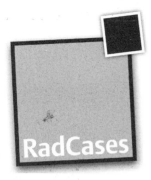

RadCases

Interventional Radiology

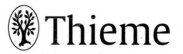

Thieme

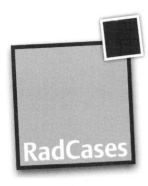

Interventional Radiology

Edited by

Hector Ferral, MD
Professor of Radiology
Section Chief, Interventional Radiology
Rush University Medical Center, Chicago
Chicago, Illinois

Jonathan Lorenz, MD
Associate Professor of Radiology
Department of Radiology
The University of Chicago
Chicago, Illinois

Series Editors

Jonathan Lorenz, MD
Associate Professor of Radiology
Department of Radiology
The University of Chicago
Chicago, Illinois

Hector Ferral, MD
Professor of Radiology
Section Chief, Interventional Radiology
Rush University Medical Center, Chicago
Chicago, Illinois

Thieme
New York • Stuttgart

Thieme Medical Publishers, Inc.
333 Seventh Ave.
New York, NY 10001

Executive Editor: Timothy Hiscock
Editorial Director: Michael Wachinger
Editorial Assistant: Adriana di Giorgio
International Production Director: Andreas Schabert
Production Editor: Heidi Grauel, Maryland Composition
Vice President, International Marketing and Sales: Cornelia Schulze
Chief Financial Officer: James W. Mitos
President: Brian D. Scanlan
Compositor: MPS Content Services
Printer: The Maple-Vail Book Manufacturing Group

Library of Congress Cataloging-in-Publication Data

Interventional radiology / edited by Hector Ferral, Jonathan Lorenz.
     p. ; cm.—(RadCases)
  Includes bibliographical references and index.
  ISBN 978-1-60406-177-2
  1. Interventional radiology—Case studies. I. Ferral, Hector. II. Lorenz, Jonathan. III. Series: RadCases.
  [DNLM: 1. Radiography, Interventional—methods—Case Reports. 2. Diagnosis, Differential—Case Reports. WN 200 I61211 2010]
  RD33.55.I5825 2010
  617′.05—dc22
                                    2009037652

Important note: Medical knowledge is ever-changing. As new research and clinical experience broaden our knowledge, changes in treatment and drug therapy may be required. The authors and editors of the material herein have consulted sources believed to be reliable in their efforts to provide information that is complete and in accord with the standards accepted at the time of publication. However, in view of the possibility of human error by the authors, editors, or publisher of the work herein or changes in medical knowledge, neither the authors, editors, nor publisher, nor any other party who has been involved in the preparation of this work, warrants that the information contained herein is in every respect accurate or complete, and they are not responsible for any errors or omissions or for the results obtained from use of such information. Readers are encouraged to confirm the information contained herein with other sources. For example, readers are advised to check the product information sheet included in the package of each drug they plan to administer to be certain that the information contained in this publication is accurate and that changes have not been made in the recommended dose or in the contraindications for administration. This recommendation is of particular importance in connection with new or infrequently used drugs.

Some of the product names, patents, and registered designs referred to in this book are in fact registered trademarks or proprietary names even though specific reference to this fact is not always made in the text. Therefore, the appearance of a name without designation as proprietary is not to be construed as a representation by the publisher that it is in the public domain.

Printed in the United States

978-1-60406-177-2

To my two sons, Manuel and Emilio, who keep me alive and happy, and to Michelle who has given me the energy and enthusiasm to see life from a different perspective.

—*Hector Ferral*

To my wife, Cynthia, for her endless love and support, and to my son, Matthew—a precious gift to me just weeks before publication of this book.

—*Jonathan Lorenz*

RadCases Series Preface

The ability to assimilate detailed information across the entire spectrum of radiology is the Holy Grail sought by those preparing for their trip to Louisville. As enthusiastic partners in the Thieme RadCases series who formerly took the examination, we understand the exhaustion and frustration shared by residents and the families of residents engaged in this quest. It has been our observation that despite ongoing efforts to improve Web-based interactive databases, residents still find themselves searching for material they can review while preparing for the radiology board examinations and remain frustrated by the fact that only a few printed guidebooks are available, which are limited in both format and image quality. Perhaps their greatest source of frustration is the inability to easily locate groups of cases across all subspecialties of radiology that are organized and tailored for their immediate study needs. Imagine being able to immediately access groups of high-quality cases to arrange study sessions, quickly extract and master information, and prepare for theme-based radiology conferences. Our goal in creating the RadCases series was to combine the popularity and portability of printed books with the adaptability, exceptional quality, and interactive features of an electronic case-based format.

The intent of the printed book is to encourage repeated priming in the use of critical information by providing a portable group of exceptional core cases that the resident can master. The best way to determine the format for these cases was to ask residents from around the country to weigh in. Overwhelmingly, the residents said that they would prefer a concise, point-by-point presentation of the Essential Facts of each case in an easy-to-read, bulleted format. Differentials are limited to a maximum of three, and the first is always the actual diagnosis. This approach is easy on exhausted eyes and provides a quick review of Pearls and Pitfalls as information is absorbed during repeated study sessions. We worked hard to choose cases that could be presented well in this format, recognizing the limitations inherent in reproducing high-quality images in print. Unlike the authors of other case-based radiology review books, we removed the guesswork by providing clear annotations and descriptions for all images. In our opinion, there is nothing worse than being unable to locate a subtle finding on a poorly reproduced image even after one knows the final diagnosis.

The electronic cases expand on the printed book and provide a comprehensive review of the entire subspecialty. Thousands of cases are strategically designed to increase the resident's knowledge by providing exposure to additional case examples—from basic to advanced—and by exploring "Aunt Minnie's," unusual diagnoses, and variability within a single diagnosis. The search engine gives the resident a fighting chance to find the Holy Grail by creating individualized, daily study lists that are not limited by factors such as radiology subsection. For example, tailor today's study list to cases involving tuberculosis and include cases in every subspecialty and every system of the body. Or study only thoracic cases, including those with links to cardiology, nuclear medicine, and pediatrics. Or study only musculoskeletal cases. The choice is yours.

As enthusiastic partners in this project, we started small and, with the encouragement, talent, and guidance of Tim Hiscock at Thieme, we have continued to raise the bar in our effort to assist residents in tackling the daunting task of assimilating massive amounts of information. We are passionate about continuing this journey, planning to expand the cases in our electronic series, adapt cases based on direct feedback from residents, and increase the features intended for board review and self-assessment. As the National Board of Medical Examiners converts the American Board of Radiology examination from an oral to an electronic format, our series will be the one best suited to meet the needs of the next generation of overworked and exhausted residents in radiology.

Jonathan Lorenz, MD
Hector Ferral, MD
Chicago, IL

Preface

The passion we both share for teaching residents serves not only as our daily motivation, but as the foundation for our academic careers and the reason we teamed up to write *Interventional Radiology*, part of the RadCases series. If you are a resident considering buying this book, you should know that it has taken us about 10 years to compile these cases, and we have used them to train our residents and fellows and to prepare them for the oral board exams. Actually, it was our residents who gave us the idea and encouragement to undertake this project after our collection of cases led to a track record of consistent success on the boards. You should also know that we remember what it was like to stand in your shoes. We remember combing through everything from review books to encyclopedias of endless information to find a way to absorb impossible amounts of knowledge in a few month-long subspecialty rotations—all the while manning our clinical responsibilities. Our frustration over the lack of concise, accurate, and comprehensive interventional radiology review materials for the oral board exam was the seed for the development of this book and, ultimately, the RadCases series.

The oral board examiner in interventional radiology wants to see competence in diagnosis, treatment options, basic technical knowledge, and clinical follow-up—all emphasized in the Essential Facts and Pearls and Pitfalls of this book. Your success depends on repeated priming of these details while reviewing a core set of cases covering the most common diagnoses and interventional procedures. This printed book makes repeated priming possible by exposing you to essential cases that are most likely to appear on the oral exam, including the gamut of vascular and nonvascular, diagnostic and interventional cases. In the home stretch, your goal should be to review core concepts while minimizing nonessential and distracting details. The electronic component consists of sortable, concise, high-resolution cases that will help you achieve this goal.

Cases 1 to 50 were authored by Hector Ferral and cases 51 to 100 were authored by Jonathan Lorenz.

Acknowledgments

We would like to thank Timothy Hiscock at Thieme Publishers for his expertise, patience, and encouragement and Adriana diGiorgio for her expert technical assistance.

Case 1

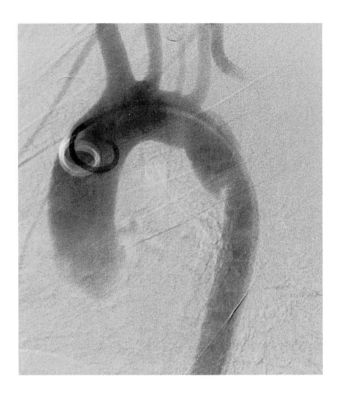

■ **Clinical Presentation**

The patient is a 27-year-old man involved in a head-on collision.

■ Imaging Findings

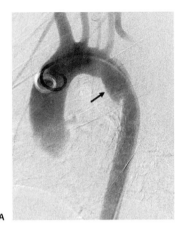
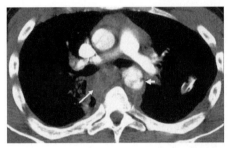

A   B

(A) Digital subtraction aortogram in the left anterior oblique (LAO) view demonstrates contour irregularity in the aortic isthmus (*arrow*). There is a separate origin of the left vertebral artery directly from the aortic arch. The finding is confirmed in the anteroposterior (AP) and right anterior oblique (RAO) views. **(B)** CT findings in aortic injury include the following: mediastinal or periaortic hematoma (*white arrow*), irregularity of the aortic lumen (*arrowhead*), hemothorax, and fractures.

■ Differential Diagnosis

- ***Traumatic injury to the aorta:*** The increase in caliber of the aortic lumen at the isthmus and the aortic wall irregularity are strong signs.
- *Ductus bump:* The contours are smooth in a ductus bump.
- *Ulcerated plaque of the aorta:* This is usually eccentric and does not enlarge the aortic lumen.

■ Essential Facts

- Blunt aortic injury is common in the setting of severe trauma.
- The most common site of injury is the aortic root. Most of these patients die at the scene.
- The most common site of aortic injury diagnosed with imaging studies is the aortic isthmus, just distal to the origin of the left subclavian artery.
- Of all patients with blunt aortic injury, ~85% die at the scene.
- Of the 10 to 15% of patients who arrive at hospital alive, 20% die of aortic rupture.

■ Additional Imaging

- Contrast-enhanced computed tomography (CT) is the study of choice for evaluation of the thoracic aorta in trauma patients.

✔ Pearls & ✗ Pitfalls

- ✔ Diagnostic aortography is still performed in several institutions.
- ✔ A high-quality aortogram is essential for the diagnosis.
- ✔ Always obtain three views (RAO, LAO, and AP).
- ✔ Look for irregularity in the contour of the aorta, especially at the isthmus; it may be subtle.
- ✔ Always review the brachiocephalic trunk and the left carotid and subclavian arteries; they are involved in 5 to 10% of cases.
- ✔ *If the CT or angiographic findings are positive, they should be reported immediately to the referring physician as this is a potentially fatal condition if not addressed immediately.*

Case 2

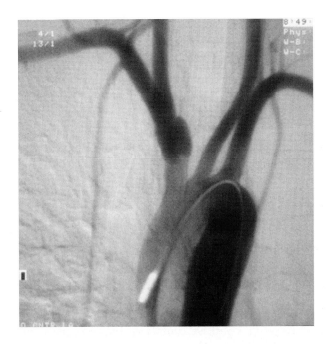

Clinical Presentation

The patient is a 22-year-old man involved in a head-on collision.

■ Imaging Findings

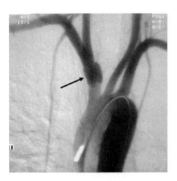

Digital subtraction aortogram in the right anterior oblique (RAO) view demonstrates contour irregularity of the right brachiocephalic artery (*arrow*). The left carotid and left subclavian arteries are of normal appearance.

■ Differential Diagnosis

- ***Blunt vascular injury of the right brachiocephalic artery:*** Enlargement of the artery and contour irregularity are key signs.
- *Aneurysm of the right brachiocephalic artery:* Aneurysms may be fusiform but do not cause the contour irregularity seen in this case.
- *Pseudoaneurysm:* This is usually seen as a saccular extravasation close to the injured site.

■ Essential Facts

- Blunt aortic injury is common in the setting of severe trauma.
- The most common site is the aortic isthmus, just distal to the origin of the left subclavian artery (88%).
- The arteries of the neck are involved in 10 to 12% of cases.
- Multirow-detector computed tomography (CT) has sensitivity of 96%, specificity of 99%, and accuracy of 99% in the diagnosis of blunt aortic trauma.
- Confirmatory arteriography is sometimes requested by the trauma surgeon.
- A two- or three-view, high-flow (30–40 mL/s) arteriogram obtained via a high-flow (6F or 7F) pigtail catheter is essential for the diagnosis.

✔ Pearls & ✗ Pitfalls

- ✔ In an arch arteriogram, always review the neck vessels.
- ✔ A high-flow aortogram in at least two views is essential for the diagnosis.
- ✔ Always review the diagnostic CT before arteriography is begun. It may guide you to a specific area that you want to evaluate.
- ✔ **If the result is positive, contact the referring physician immediately. These are critical lesions.**

Case 3

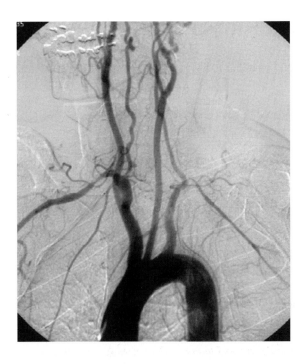

■ Clinical Presentation

A 67-year-old woman presents with weakness of the left arm, claudication of the jaw, and headaches.

■ Imaging Findings

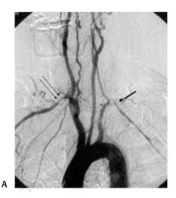
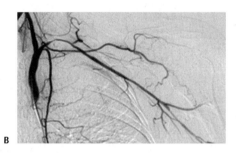
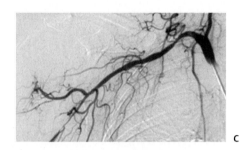

A   B   C

(A) Digital subtraction aortogram in the left anterior oblique view demonstrates a smooth decrease in caliber of the right subclavian artery (*double arrow*) and a severe smooth decrease in caliber of the left mid and distal portions of the subclavian artery (*arrow*). The thoracic aorta is normal. **(B,C)** Selective injections of the left **(B)** and right **(C)** subclavian arteries depict the vascular changes in a more precise fashion.

■ Differential Diagnosis

- **Giant cell arteritis:** The findings are consistent with giant cell arteritis. The patient's age supports this possibility.
- *Takayasu's arteritis:* The angiographic findings fit, but the patient's age does not support this diagnosis.
- *Fibromuscular dysplasia:* Good option. This disease process can involve the carotid, iliac, and renal arteries; however, it is unusual to see subclavian involvement, as in this case.

■ Essential Facts

- Giant cell arteritis is a generalized vasculitis of the medium-size and large arteries.
- It is the most common primary vasculitis in persons older than 50 years.
- It is more common in women.
- Commonly involved arteries include the aortic arch and extracranial carotid arteries.
- Characteristically, histology demonstrates granulomas.

✔ Pearls & ✘ Pitfalls

- ✔ **This condition is considered a medical emergency. If it is left untreated, there is a high risk for visual loss.**
- ✔ The treatment is medical with steroids.
- ✔ Endovascular management or surgery is not indicated when the disease is active.
- ✔ Disease activity can be monitored with the erythrocyte sedimentation rate and C-reactive protein levels.
- ✘ Angiographically, giant cell arteritis is identical to Takayasu's arteritis. The differential diagnosis depends on the patient's age. If the patient is younger than 30 years, Takayasu's arteritis is the most likely diagnosis.

Case 4

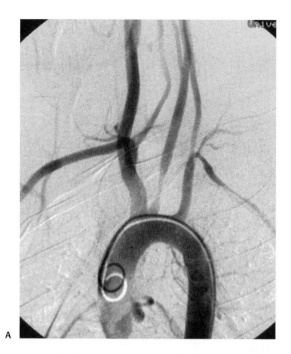

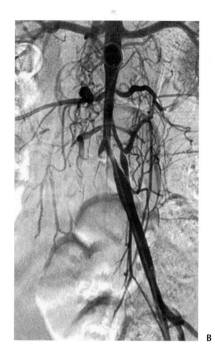

A

B

■ **Clinical Presentation**

The patient is a 13-year-old girl with a diagnosis of "vascular disease."

■ Imaging Findings

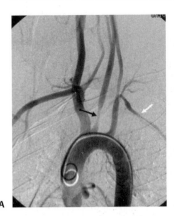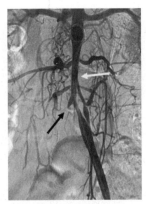

A   B

(A) Digital subtraction aortogram in the left anterior oblique view demonstrates a smooth decrease in caliber of the left common carotid artery (*black arrow*) and diffuse smooth stenosis of the left subclavian artery (*white arrow*). **(B)** The distal aorta shows smooth tapering below the renal arteries (*white arrow*). There is marked hypertrophy of the lumbar arteries. The right common iliac artery is occluded (*black arrow*).

■ Differential Diagnosis

- ***Takayasu's arteritis:*** The findings are consistent with Takayasu's arteritis. The patient's age supports this possibility.
- *Giant cell arteritis:* The angiographic findings fit, but the patient's age does not support this diagnosis.
- *Fibromuscular dysplasia (FMD):* Good option. This disease process can involve the carotid, iliac, and renal arteries; however, it is unusual to see vessel occlusion in FMD.

■ Essential Facts

- The preferred term is *obliterative brachiocephalic arteritis.*
- The disease is divided into a systemic phase and a late occlusive phase.
- It occurs in all races and age groups but is more common in women in the 2nd and 3rd decades of life.
- Cerebral ischemia is the most threatening complication.

Type 1	Aortic arch and great vessels
Type 2	Distal thoracic and abdominal aorta
Type 3	Aortic arch and abdominal aorta
Type 4	Any type + pulmonary arteries

✔ Pearls & ✘ Pitfalls

- ✔ Angiography shows long, smooth stenotic segments of the medium-size and large arteries.
- ✔ Four types have been described. Type 3, the most common, involves the aortic arch and abdominal aorta.
- ✔ Management is with steroids.
- ✔ Endovascular or surgical intervention is not recommended when the disease is in an active phase.
- ✔ Long-term patency rates after endovascular therapy are low.

Case 5

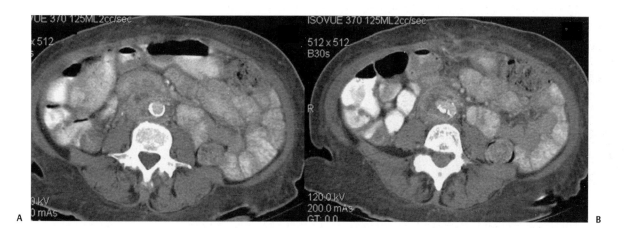

■ Clinical Presentation

The patient is a 68-year-old woman with chronic renal failure who is on dialysis.

Further Work-up

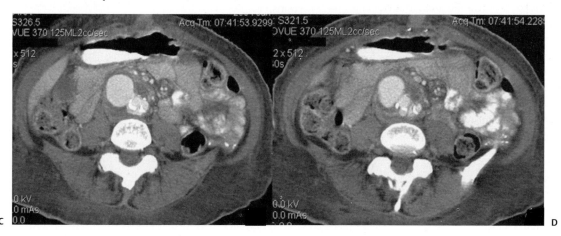

Image obtained 15 days later.

■ Imaging Findings

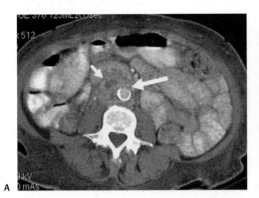 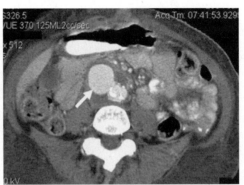

(A) Axial image of the first contrast-enhanced computed tomographic (CT) scan shows a large area of soft-tissue density and irregular areas of decreased density surrounding the distal abdominal aorta and extending into the proximal portions of the iliac arteries (*white arrowhead*). These findings are consistent with periaortic inflammation. Note the discontinuity of the calcification of the aortic wall (*white arrow*). **(B)** Axial image of the contrast-enhanced CT scan obtained 2 weeks later demonstrates a bright, well-defined, contained saccular area of contrast enhancement in the region previously seen as a periaortic soft-tissue density (*white arrow*).

■ Differential Diagnosis

- **Mycotic aneurysm:** The findings show a rapidly developing saccular aneurysm of the lower abdominal aorta. The patient had a fever and an elevated white blood cell count. With this clinical picture, mycotic aneurysm is the first diagnostic possibility.
- *Saccular, noninfected aortic aneurysm:* This is unlikely because of the evolution on imaging.
- *Aortic pseudoaneurysm:* This is unlikely because the patient has no history of trauma and the evolution on imaging does not match the diagnosis.

✔ Pearls & ✘ Pitfalls

- ✔ Mycotic aneurysms account for 1 to 3% of all aortic aneurysms.
- ✔ Ninety-three percent of mycotic aneurysms are saccular, eccentric, or lobulated aneurysms.
- ✔ Always look at the aortic calcifications! The wall of the mycotic aneurysm is not calcified.
- ✔ Contrast-enhanced CT may reveal masslike periaortic inflammation, fluid, pneumatosis, or rupture.

■ Essential Facts

- Primary aortic infection generally begins with bacteremia from a remote portal of entry.
- Common organisms include *Staphylococcus aureus*, *Salmonella*, and *Streptococcus pneumoniae*.
- Infection within the aortic wall leads to aortic degeneration and rapid growth of an aneurysm.
- Predisposing factors are atherosclerosis and immune deficiency (transplant or AIDS).
- The condition is potentially fatal if left untreated.

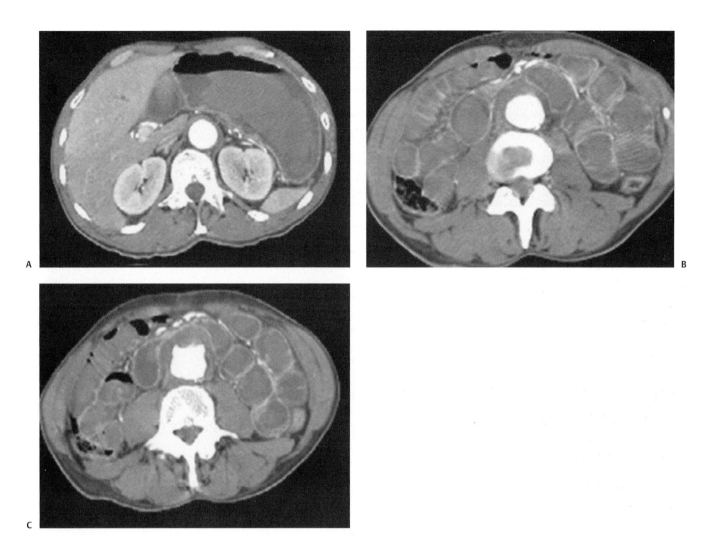

Clinical Presentation

The patient is a 75-year-old man with history of back pain treated with nonsteroidal anti-inflammatory drugs.

■ Imaging Findings

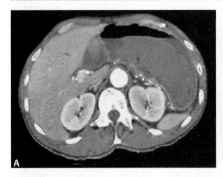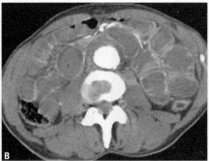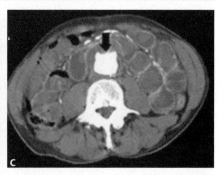

(A–C) Selected axial images of a contrast-enhanced computed tomographic (CT) scan of the abdomen demonstrate material of increased density within the lumen of the stomach **(A)** and small bowel **(B)**. This is consistent with a massive amount of blood throughout the gastrointestinal tract. **(C)** Enlargement of the aortic lumen with contour irregularity (*arrow*).

■ Differential Diagnosis

- **Abdominal aortic aneurysm with primary aortoenteric fistula (AEF):** The combination of an abdominal aortic aneurysm (AAA) and blood in the gastrointestinal tract makes primary AEF the first diagnostic possibility.
- *Massive gastrointestinal (GI) bleeding from another source*

■ Essential Facts

- Primary AEF with massive GI bleeding is a very rare presentation of AAA (0.7% of AAAs).
- It is a communication between the infrarenal aorta and the 3rd or 4th portion of the duodenum.
- The aneurysms are infected in ~30% of cases.
- Common microorganisms are *Staphylococcus aureus* and *S. epidermidis*.
- Secondary AEF is a communication between the bowel and a prosthetic graft.

✔ Pearls & ✘ Pitfalls

- ✔ The classic triad of GI bleeding, sepsis, and abdominal pain is seen in < 30% of cases.
- ✔ CT findings include ectopic gas, focal thickening of the bowel wall, periaortic fluid, and perigraft soft tissue.
- ✔ Treatment is surgical, usually with closure of the aorta and extra-anatomical bypass.
- ✔ Mortality is very high, ranging between 30 and 60%.

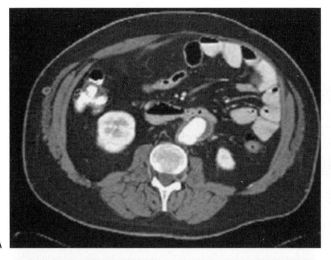

A

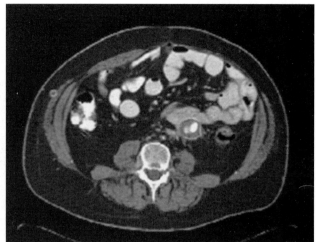

B

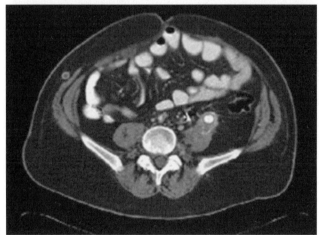

C

■ Clinical Presentation

The patient is a 38-year-old man with abdominal pain and fever.

■ Imaging Findings

- Selected axial images of a contrast-enhanced computed tomographic (CT) scan of the abdomen demonstrate fluid density surrounding an aorto-bifemoral bypass graft from the upper cuts to the pelvic cuts.

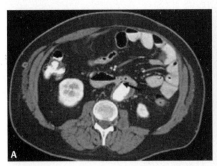 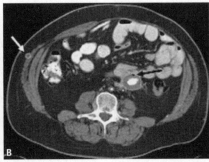 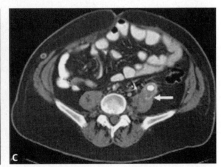

(A,B) Figures show loss of the tissue separation plane between the fluid surrounding the graft and the 3rd portion of the duodenum; a small collection of air is also identified (*arrow*). Incidentally, an occluded axillofemoral bypass is identified within the soft tissues on the right side (*white arrow,* **B**). **(C)** The perigraft fluid extends caudally to the upper pelvis and seems to involve the left psoas muscle (*white arrow*).

■ Differential Diagnosis

- **Aorto-bifemoral graft infection, occluded axillofemoral bypass:** The presence of gas and fluid around the aorto-bifemoral graft strongly indicates graft infection.
- *Noninfected perigraft fluid:* This is unlikely. It is common ~2 to 3 weeks after surgery.
- *Secondary aortoenteric (AEF) fistula with perigraft infection:* This has to be in the differential diagnosis; however, there is no history of bleeding.

■ Essential Facts

- **Prompt diagnosis and treatment are essential**.
- Contrast-enhanced CT is the imaging technique of choice for the evaluation of graft infection.
- CT-guided aspiration of perigraft fluid is useful to identify the microorganism.
- *Staphylococcus aureus* is the most prevalent pathogen in perigraft infections.
- Secondary AEF is a communication between the bowel and a prosthetic graft.
- Although rare, secondary AEF is more common than primary AEF. The incidence ranges between 0.4 and 2.0%.

✔ Pearls & ✘ Pitfalls

- ✔ The presence of air and fluid around a prosthetic graft is considered to be normal up to 6 to 7 weeks after graft implantation. After 6 to 7 weeks, gas surrounding the graft is indicative of infection but does not confirm an association with AEF.
- ✔ CT findings indicative of AEF include visualization of a graft in close proximity to the bowel lumen and active extravasation. Indirect CT findings suggestive of AEF include effacement of the perigraft fat plane, perigraft soft tissue, and thickening of the bowel wall adjacent to the graft.
- ✔ Endovascular grafts can also present with signs of infection.

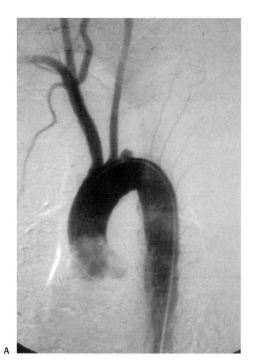

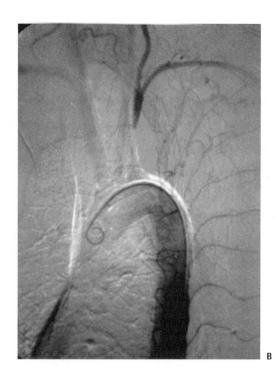

Clinical Presentation

The patient is a 57-year-old left-handed carpenter with claudication of the arm and dizziness.

■ Imaging Findings

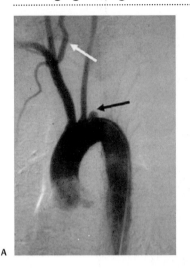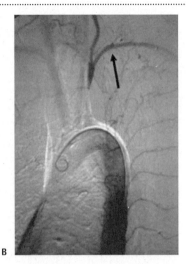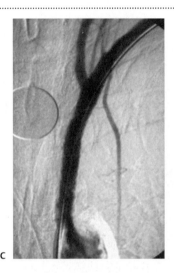

A   B   C

(A) Selected image from a digital subtraction arteriogram (DSA) of the aortic arch in a steep left anterior oblique projection demonstrates a patent right brachiocephalic trunk and left carotid artery. The right vertebral artery is prominent (*white arrow*). The left subclavian artery is occluded, and only a small stump is visualized (*black arrow*). **(B)** A later frame of the same DSA run shows delayed retrograde opacification of the left vertebral artery and flow into the distal left subclavian artery (*arrow*). **(C)** Result after endovascular placement of a subclavian artery stent.

■ Differential Diagnosis

- **Left subclavian artery occlusion with subclavian steal (SS) syndrome**
- *SS phenomenon*

■ Essential Facts

- The term *SS syndrome* should be reserved for retrograde vertebral artery flow associated with transient neurologic symptoms related to cerebral ischemia.
- The term *SS phenomenon* refers to asymptomatic retrograde flow in the vertebral artery.
- SS phenomenon is more common on the left side (4:1).

✔ Pearls & ✘ Pitfalls

- ✔ **If you see films showing subclavian artery occlusion, you should promptly ask if the patient is symptomatic.**
- ✔ Commonly symptomatic. If asymptomatic, there is no indication for treatment.
- ✔ Symptoms that occur (dizziness, unsteadiness, vertigo, visual changes) are most typically related to vertebrobasilar and posterior cerebral circulation ischemia.
- ✔ Arm claudication and pain at rest indicate a component of arm ischemia.

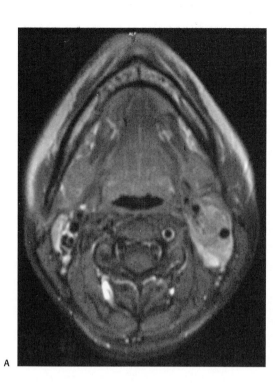

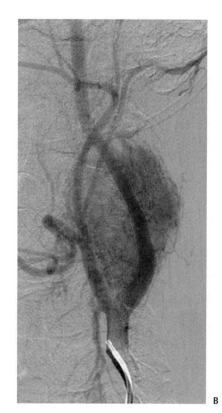

A

B

■ Clinical Presentation

The patient is a 23-year-old woman with neck mass and palpitations.

■ Imaging Findings

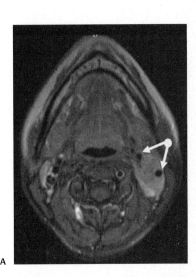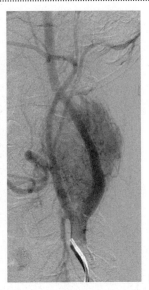

A   B

(A) Selected axial image of a T2-weighted magnetic resonance imaging study at the level of the upper neck showing a smooth soft-tissue mass at the carotid bifurcation. The mass separates the two carotid arteries (*arrows*). **(B)** Selected image from a digital subtraction arteriogram of the left carotid artery with the catheter selectively placed in the left common carotid artery. Contrast injection confirms the presence of a large, hypervascular mass between the left internal and external carotid arteries.

■ Differential Diagnosis

• **Carotid body glomus tumor**
• The image is fairly typical, but you may want to consider neurogenic tumor from the carotid sheath contents.

■ Essential Facts

• These tumors may be sporadic or hereditary.
• Transmission of hereditary tumors is autosomal-dominant.
• Most of these tumors are benign; only 6 to 12% are malignant.

✔ Pearls & ✗ Pitfalls

✔ Carotid angiography is indicated to evaluate multiplicity, hypervascularity, and the possibility of presurgical embolization.
✔ The blood supply for carotid body tumors is typically from the ascending pharyngeal artery.
✔ Clinically, these tumors are mobile in the lateral plane, but not in the craniocaudal direction (Fontaine's sign) as they transmit the pulse; they may cause dysphagia, hoarseness, and neural deficits (cranial nerves IX–XII).
✔ The tumors may accumulate norepinephrine and cause hypertension, palpitations, flushing, and perspiration.

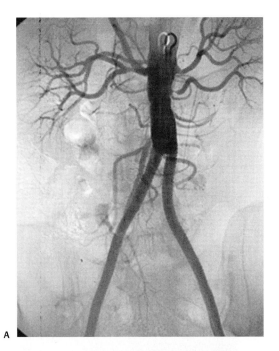

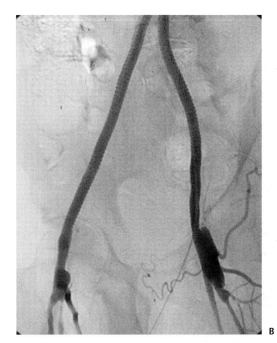

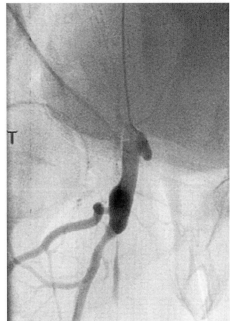

■ Clinical Presentation

The patient is a 73-year-old veteran with a history of vascular surgery and a cold right foot.

■ Imaging Findings

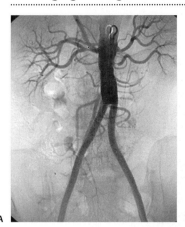 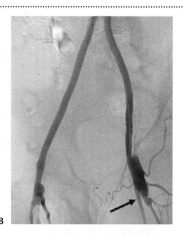 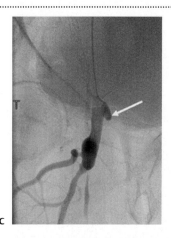

A   B   C

(A) Selected image from a nonselective digital subtraction arteriogram of the abdominal aorta showing patent renal arteries, an accessory left lower renal artery that has an ostial stenosis, and a patent aorto-bifemoral graft with an end-to end anastomosis to the aorta. **(B)** Patent right and left limbs of the aorto-bifemoral graft. Post-surgical changes are identified in the left limb of the graft at the femoral anastomosis. The takeoff of a left femoral–popliteal graft is identified (*arrow*). The takeoff of a right femoral–popliteal graft is not identified. **(C)** Image obtained after selective injection into the right limb of the aorto-bifemoral graft in a right anterior oblique view showing a small stump corresponding to the takeoff of the occluded right femoral–popliteal graft.

■ Differential Diagnosis

- *Occluded femoral–popliteal graft causing acute limb ischemia*
- *Severe peripheral vascular disease*

■ Essential Facts

- Patients with acute limb ischemia need to be evaluated clinically. Clinical categories include the following:
- 1. Viable. Not threatened. Good candidates for lytic therapy.
- 2a. Acutely threatened. Slow capillary return, minimal sensory loss (toes), no muscle weakness. No Doppler arterial signals. Good candidates for lytic therapy.
- 2b. Immediately threatened. Salvaged if immediately revascularized. More sensory loss, mild-to-moderate weakness. No Doppler arterial signal. Lytic therapy only if patient is a poor surgical candidate.
- 3. Irreversible. Major tissue loss or permanent nerve damage. No capillary return, profound sensory loss, paralysis, and no Doppler signals (arterial or venous). These patients should go to surgery.

✔ Pearls & ✘ Pitfalls

- ✔ In catheter-directed thrombolysis, an infusion catheter is embedded within a thrombus.
- ✔ Better results are expected if the thrombosis is acute (< 14 days).
- ✔ A common drug is the recombinant tissue–type plasminogen activator (rt-PA) alteplase (Activase, Genentech, South San Francisco, CA). The dose ranges from 0.25 to 2 mg/h.
- ✔ Patients need to be monitored with bleeding precautions.
- ✔ Lytic therapy is absolutely contraindicated in patients with active bleeding, recent stroke, recent surgery, or a brain tumor.

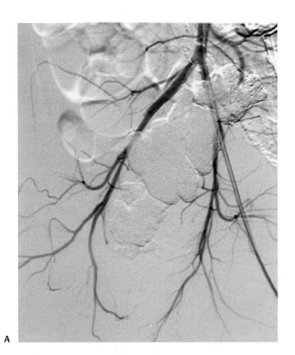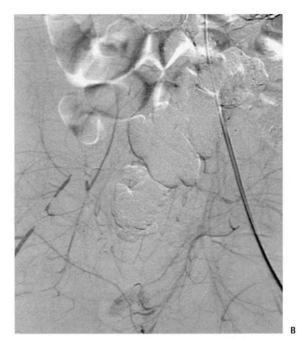

A   B

■ Clinical Presentation

The patient is a 7-month-old baby with tetralogy of Fallot.

■ Imaging Findings

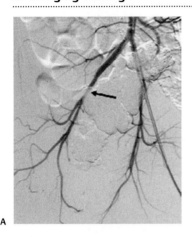
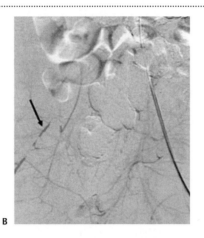
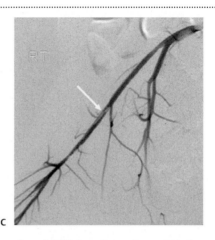

A   B   C

(A) Nonselective digital subtraction arteriogram (DSA) of the iliac arteries showing occlusion of the right external iliac artery. Only the right internal iliac artery is opacified (*arrow*). **(B)** Late image of the same pelvic DSA showing delayed opacification of a partially occluded right external iliac artery (*arrow*). **(C)** Selected image from a DSA after pulse spray thrombolysis showing a patent external iliac artery with mild residual stenosis, which corresponds to a small residual thrombus (*white arrow*).

■ Differential Diagnosis

- ***Acute occlusion of the right external iliac artery secondary to arterial catheterization:*** Note that there are no collaterals. This fact supports an acute process.
- *Iliac artery dissection:* Arteriography after thrombolysis does not show dissection.
- *Acute embolism of the right iliac artery:* The possibility of embolism may be considered because the patient has heart disease.

■ Essential Facts

- Small children are not good candidates for long-term infusion of lytic therapy. Systemic thrombolysis by infusion of the drug via the vein is preferred.
- If the thrombosis needs to be managed urgently, a fast method such as the pulse spray technique may be attempted.
- Mechanical thrombectomy devices can be used, but with caution, in pediatric patients. They may be too large for the small arteries of children.

✔ Pearls & ✗ Pitfalls

- ✔ Use real-time ultrasound guidance for arterial and venous access in pediatric patients.
- ✔ The dose of the recombinant tissue–type plasminogen activator (rt-PA) alteplase (Activase, Genentech, South San Francisco, CA) in children ranges between 0.25 and 1 mg/h.

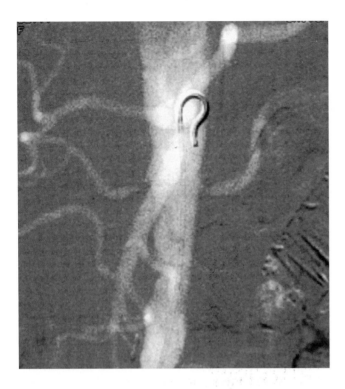

■ **Clinical Presentation**

The patient is a 69-year-old woman, an ex-smoker, who is not diabetic and has a serum creatinine level of 2.5 mg/dL.

■ Imaging Findings

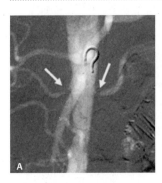
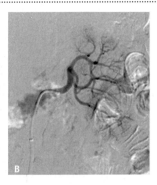
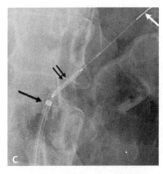
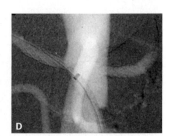

(A) Nonselective digital subtraction arteriogram (DSA) of the abdominal aorta with carbon dioxide shows severe ostial stenosis of both renal arteries (*white arrows*). The patient is a candidate for stent placement with carbon dioxide used as a contrast agent. **(B)** During stent placement, the lesion should be crossed carefully, heparin should be administered, and angiography should be used to rule out dissection or distal thrombosis. A vasodilator should be administered intra-arterially to prevent severe spasm. **(C)** A stent should be selected that is appropriate for the size of the artery and length of the lesion (*double arrows*). A guiding catheter (*black arrow*) is useful to provide support for stent placement. The guide wire should always be within the field of view to avoid distal arterial perforation (*white arrow*). **(D)** An arteriogram should be obtained after deployment to confirm successful stent placement.

■ Differential Diagnosis

- **Bilateral renal artery ostial stenosis, most probably atherosclerotic**
- *Fibromuscular dysplasia:* The ostial location of the stenotic areas and the patient's age do not support this possibility.
- *Vasculitis:* This is also a possibility; however, the clinical presentation and the angiographic appearance do not support vasculitis.

■ Essential Facts

- Renal artery revascularization is indicated in patients with documented renal artery stenosis and a significant sign such as hypertension, flash pulmonary edema, or an elevated serum creatinine level.
- Patients with a serum creatinine level > 3.0 mg/dL have a worse prognosis and a poor response to treatment.

✔ Pearls & ✘ Pitfalls

- ✔ Atherosclerotic renal artery ostial stenosis is better treated with primary stent placement.
- ✔ Balloon-expandable stents are preferred for this location as their placement is very precise.

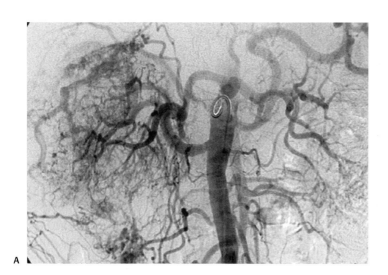

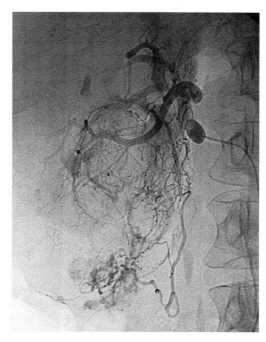

A   B

■ Clinical Presentation

The patient is a 56-year-old woman with back pain.

■ Imaging Findings

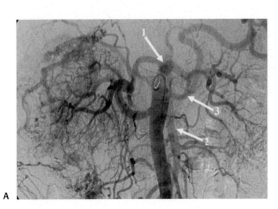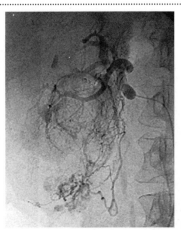

(A) Nonselective digital subtraction arteriogram of the abdominal aorta in an anteroposterior projection demonstrates a large, hypervascular right kidney. A mass per se is not well defined in the image. The image also demonstrates the celiac trunk (*arrow 1*), superior mesenteric artery (*arrow 2*), and left renal artery (*arrow 3*). (B) Selected image from a selective balloon occlusion arteriogram of the right kidney from the same patient demonstrates a large, hypervascular mass in the lower pole. No direct arteriovenous communication, reflux of contrast, or extravasation is identified.

■ Differential Diagnosis

- *Renal cell carcinoma:* The mass is hypervascular and shows a heterogeneous pattern.
- *Oncocytoma:* The angiographic picture does not support oncocytoma, which is usually well circumscribed and (occasionally) supplied by branching arteries with a "spoked wheel" configuration. The vascularity in the present case is irregular and random.
- *Angiomyolipoma:* Additional imaging with computed tomography is useful. This tumor usually shows a large lipid component.

✔ Pearls & ✘ Pitfalls

- ✔ Careful monitoring of the vital signs is important as ethanol-induced arrhythmia and pulmonary artery pressure changes may occur during injection.

■ Essential Facts

- The best treatment for renal cell carcinoma is surgical removal.
- Large tumors may be difficult to resect.
- Some urologists favor alcohol ablation of the involved kidney before surgery. The purpose of this procedure is to decrease intraoperative bleeding.
- Ethanol ablation may also be used in patients with unresectable tumors as a palliative measure.
- The patient shown in this case underwent presurgical ethanol ablation of a right-sided renal cell carcinoma.

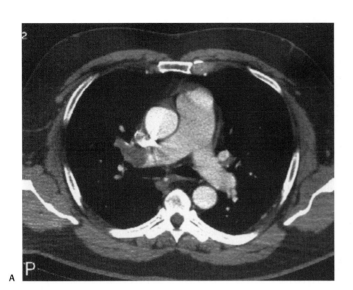

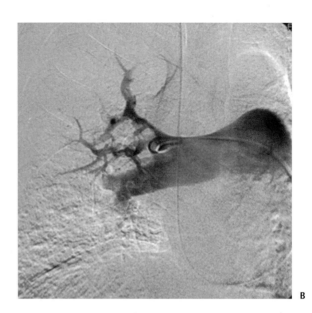

■ Clinical Presentation

The patient is a 58-year-old man with shortness of breath.

■ Imaging Findings

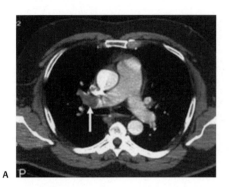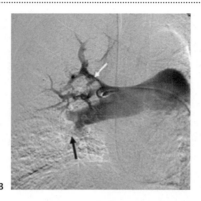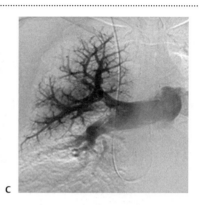

A   P   B   C

(A) Image from a contrast-enhanced computed tomographic (CT) scan at the level of the pulmonary artery bifurcation demonstrating a large filling defect within the lumen of the right pulmonary artery (*arrow*). No other significant imaging findings are demonstrated. **(B)** Image of a selective right pulmonary arteriogram. There is a large filling defect within the superior segmental branch (*white arrow*). Abrupt occlusion (*black arrow*) is seen in the two lower branches. **(C)** Image of a selective right pulmonary arteriogram 48 hours after treatment with catheter-directed thrombolysis. The pulmonary artery is now patent with no detectable filling defects.

■ Differential Diagnosis

- ***Acute massive embolism of the right pulmonary artery***
- *Intravascular tumor:* An intravascular tumor can mimic acute pulmonary embolism (PE). The clinical history and evidence of tumor at another site or locally help make the diagnosis.
- *Chronic pulmonary embolism:* This condition usually presents with diffuse irregularity of the pulmonary arteries but no large filling defects.

■ Essential Facts

- The principal criterion by which acute PE is characterized as massive is systemic arterial hypotension.
- Massive PE carries a very high mortality rate, and a rapid diagnosis is crucial to initiate therapy.
- Pulmonary CT angiography has virtually replaced lung scanning for the diagnosis of PE.
- Chest CT can detect massive emboli and right ventricular (RV) enlargement (patients with RV enlargement are at risk for early death).

- Therapeutic options in massive PE include the following: systemic anticoagulation, systemic thrombolysis, endovascular mechanical thrombectomy, endovascular clot fragmentation with lytic therapy, catheter-directed thrombolysis, and surgical embolectomy.
- Currently, the drug of choice for catheter-directed thrombolysis is alteplase (Activase, Genentech, South San Francisco, CA) at doses ranging between 0.25 and 2 mg/h.

✔ Pearls & ✘ Pitfalls

- ✔ Criteria for aggressive intervention in patients with PE include hypotension, RV failure, and the need for intubation.

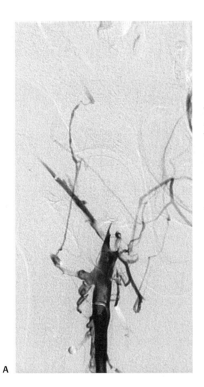

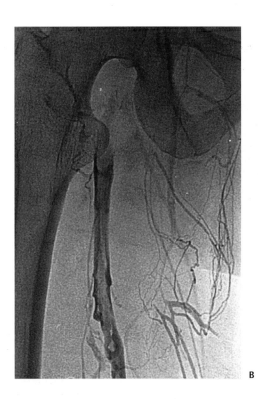

A

B

Clinical Presentation

The patient is a 57-year-old woman with a deficiency of protein C. She presents with acute swelling of a lower extremity.

■ Imaging Findings

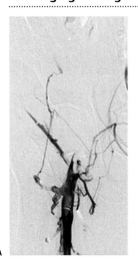
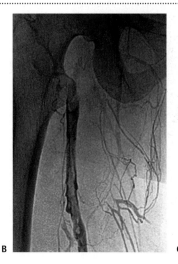
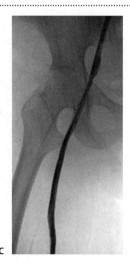

A   B   C

(A) Selected image of a lower extremity venogram demonstrates irregular filling defects within the lumen of the femoral vein, occlusion of the common femoral vein, and lack of opacification of the iliac vein. **(B)** Selected image of a femoral venogram from the same patient demonstrates a large filling defect within the lumen of the femoral vein. **(C)** Selected image of a lower extremity venogram after successful lytic therapy with alteplase (Activase, Genentech, South San Francisco, CA) at a dose of 1 mg/h. The femoral vein is now patent and free of thrombus. The external iliac vein is opacified, and no thrombus is identified.

■ Differential Diagnosis

- *Acute iliofemoral deep vein thrombosis (DVT):* The presence of large filling defects within the lumen of the vein and the lack of extensive collaterals suggest an acute process.
- *Chronic deep vein thrombosis:* This is usually seen as small channels with the development of large collaterals.
- *Traumatic venous injury:* The images could represent venous trauma; however, the large endoluminal filling defects and the lack of a history argue against this possibility.

■ Essential Facts

- The accepted management for DVT is systemic anticoagulation.
- Long-term benefits of catheter-directed thrombolysis in the management of patients with iliofemoral DVT have not been documented in prospective randomized trials.
- Catheter-directed thrombolysis is a therapeutic option in patients with DVT, severe symptoms, and no response to systemic anticoagulation.
- The catheter-directed technique appears to be most effective.
- Doses of alteplase doses range between 0.25 and 2 mg/h.

✔ Pearls & ✘ Pitfalls

- ✔ The use of strict eligibility criteria has improved the safety and acceptability of this treatment.
- ✔ Careful patient evaluation and the exclusion of major contraindications to lytic therapy are of extreme importance to avoid complications.
- ✔ The optimal drug, dose, and route of administration have yet to be determined.

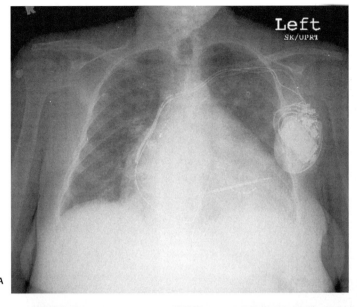

A

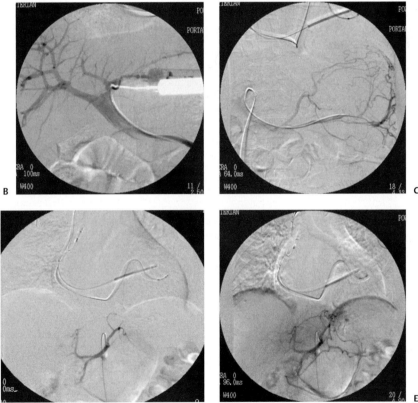

B

C

D

E

■ Clinical Presentation

A 51-year-old woman with a history of hypertension, dilated cardiomyopathy, and right-sided heart failure presents to the emergency department with upper gastrointestinal (GI) bleeding. Placement of a transjugular intrahepatic portosystemic shunt (TIPS) is requested.

■ Imaging Findings

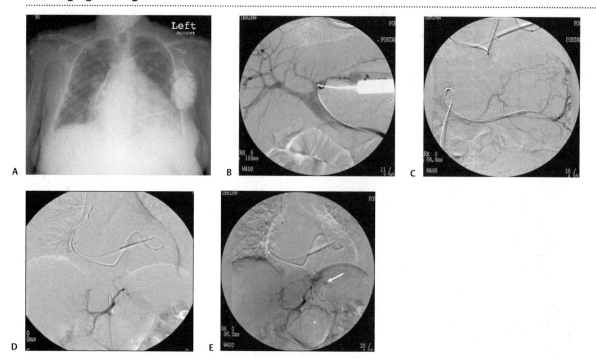

(A) Posteroanterior film of the chest shows cardiomegaly and a pacemaker inserted via the left subclavian vein with its leads in the proper position. **(B)** Image from a direct portogram performed via a catheter inserted percutaneously through the left portal vein shows opacification of the intrahepatic portal branches. There is no retrograde flow into esophageal or gastric varices. **(C)** Image from a direct splenic venogram. The catheter is placed in the most lateral aspect of the splenic vein. There is no flow into gastric or esophageal varices. There is opacification of the short gastric veins, which drain into the portal vein via the left gastric vein. **(D)** Image from a selective arteriogram of the celiac trunk. The left gastric artery, left hepatic artery, and gastroduodenal artery are visualized **(E)** Late frame from the same arteriogram shows a persistent collection of contrast in the gastric fundus (*white arrow*), consistent with active bleeding.

■ Differential Diagnosis

- ***Gastric ulcer with active bleeding:*** The angiographic findings clearly show a source of active bleeding after injection of the celiac trunk.
- *Postsinusoidal portal hypertension*: This is not a good option. The patient was carefully evaluated, and no esophageal or gastric varices were demonstrated. You should look for another source of bleeding and not proceed with TIPS placement.
- *Posthepatic portal hypertension secondary to heart failure*: This is a good possibility; however, the direct portogram and splenic venogram did not disclose signs of portal hypertension.

■ Essential Facts

- The diagnosis is active gastric bleeding, most probably from a gastric ulcer.
- This patient required embolization of the left gastric artery, not a TIPS.
- The most important lesson from this case is that you should not act only as a technician. You should have knowledge of the anatomy and physiology of the area of interest and decide what is the best intervention for a given patient. If you have no evidence of portal hypertension, you really should not proceed with TIPS placement.

✔ Pearls & ✘ Pitfalls

✔ Patients with known portal hypertension and GI bleeding require a very careful work-up. If evidence of severe portal hypertension is not found, decompression of the portal system will not solve the problem. You should be alert to other possible causes of GI bleeding in these patients.

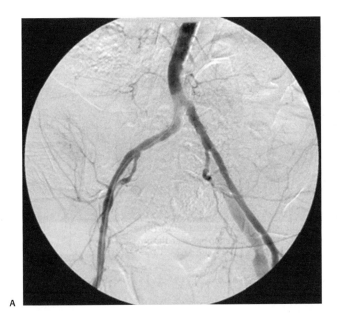
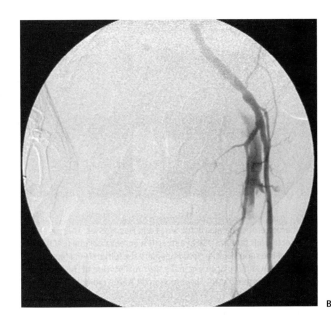

A   B

■ Clinical Presentation

The patient is a 66-year-old woman with end-stage renal disease and history of left femoral dialysis catheter placement.

■ Imaging Findings

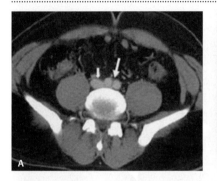
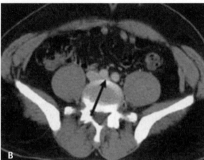
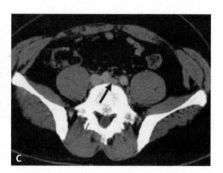

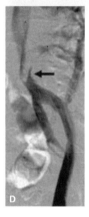
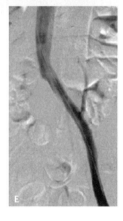

(A) Selected image from a contrast-enhanced computed tomographic (CT) scan of the pelvis at the aortic bifurcation demonstrates the aortic bifurcation (*arrow*) and inferior vena cava (*arrowhead*). (B) Selected image from a contrast-enhanced CT scan of the pelvis demonstrates compression of the left iliac vein by the right iliac artery (*arrow*). (C) Selected image from a contrast-enhanced CT scan of the pelvis demonstrates thrombus within the left iliac vein (*arrow*). (D) Selected image from a left iliac venogram after lytic therapy. The left iliac vein is patent. There is reflux of contrast into the internal iliac vein and a large lumbar collateral. Extrinsic compression of the left common iliac vein by the right iliac artery is demonstrated (*arrow*). (E) Selected image from a left iliac venogram after placement of a Wallstent (Boston Scientific, Natick, MA). The left iliac vein is now widely patent.

■ Differential Diagnosis

- ***May–Thurner syndrome (MTS) causing deep vein thrombosis (DVT):*** This is a classic case of compression of the left iliac vein by the right common iliac artery.
- *Deep vein thrombosis:* The CT scan shows thrombus within the left iliac vein; however, you should identify the compression by the artery and mention it.

■ Essential Facts

- MTS is compression of the left iliac vein by the right iliac artery.
- MTS usually presents with isolated left lower extremity DVT or symptomatic left lower extremity swelling.
- The venous compression is usually managed with placement of a self-expandable stent.

✔ Pearls & ✘ Pitfalls

- ✔ MTS should be included in the differential diagnosis of patients with isolated left-sided DVT.

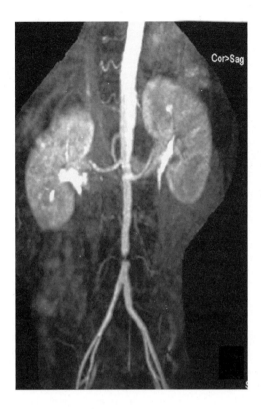

■ Clinical Presentation

The patient is a 40-year-old woman with severe claudication.

■ Imaging Findings

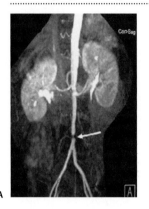
A

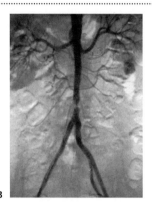
B

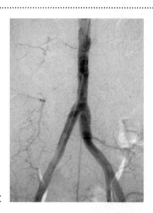
C

(A) Selected image from a contrast-enhanced magnetic resonance angiogram (MRA) of the aorta and iliac arteries demonstrating a severe distal aortic stenosis (*arrow*). **(B)** Selected image from a digital subtraction arteriogram (DSA) of the aorta and iliac arteries demonstrating severe stenosis in the distal aorta. Excellent correlation with MRA findings. **(C)** Selected image from a DSA of the aorta and iliac arteries after stent placement. No residual aortic stenosis is identified.

■ Differential Diagnosis

- ***Focal atherosclerotic stenosis in the distal aorta:*** The lesion is very suggestive of an atherosclerotic lesion. It is a focal, concentric lesion.
- *Takayasu's arteritis:* The images could represent Takayasu's arteritis. However, the patient's age does not entirely fit this diagnosis; Takayasu's arteritis is more frequent in women between 20 and 30 years of age. The arterial involvement in Takayasu's arteritis is usually more extensive and characterized by smoothly tapered narrowing. The clinical history is also important here. The woman in this case was a smoker.
- *Giant cell arteritis:* This disease entity rarely involves the aorta.

■ Essential Facts

- Short, focal atherosclerotic lesions are ideal for endovascular management.
- Excellent results can be achieved with either balloon angioplasty or stent placement.
- The 3-year patency can be as high as 85% after endovascular management.
- Balloon-expandable stents are ideal for this application.

✔ Pearls & ✘ Pitfalls

- ✔ If the angiographic findings are not diagnostic, pressures can be measured across the stenosis. A systolic pressure gradient > 10 mm Hg at rest is considered to be diagnostic of a hemodynamically significant lesion.

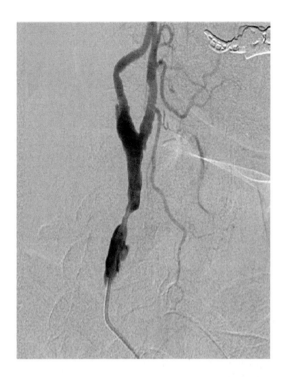

Clinical Presentation

The patient is a 58-year-old man with history of head and neck cancer.

■ Imaging Findings

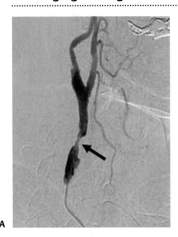 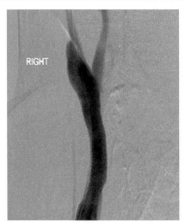

A   B

(A) Image from a selective digital subtraction arteriogram (DSA) of the right common carotid artery demonstrates a concentric, short, relatively smooth stenosis of the mid right common carotid artery. Mild irregularity of the right internal carotid artery is also noted. The right external carotid artery is patent. (B) Selected image from a DSA of the right common carotid artery after stent placement.

■ Differential Diagnosis

- **Radiation arteritis of the right common carotid artery:** Smooth, focal stenotic lesions in unusual sites strongly suggest radiation arteritis. The clinical history is important; this patient had undergone radiation therapy for a neck tumor 20 years prior.
- *Atherosclerotic stenosis of the carotid artery:* The image may correspond; however, atherosclerotic stenosis of the carotid artery usually involves the part of the internal carotid artery that is just above the bifurcation.
- *Giant cell arteritis:* The patient's age and sex are suggestive; however, the images do not support this possibility because the angiographic findings in giant cell arteritis are usually more diffuse and not as localized as those in the present case.

■ Essential Facts

- Radiation-induced vascular injury is a well-known phenomenon.
- Radiation injury rarely occurs with < 5000 rad.
- The initial presentation may occur 1 to 30 years after radiation therapy.

✔ Pearls & ✘ Pitfalls

- ✔ The diagnosis is supported by the clinical history and unusual location of the lesions.
- ✔ Placement of a self-expandable stent is a therapeutic option for patients with radiation-induced arteritis of the carotid arteries.
- ✔ Patients who undergo stent placement for this indication require periodic sonographic follow-up because intimal hyperplasia tends to develop in the treated areas.

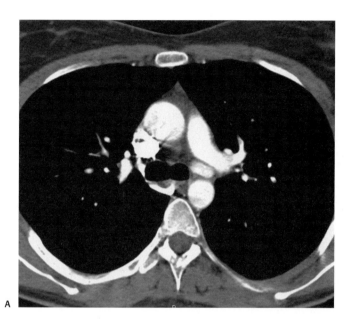

A

Clinical Presentation

The patient is a 40-year-old woman with history of motor vehicle accident 20 years prior.

Further Work-up

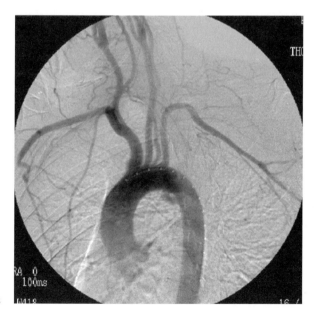

B

■ Imaging Findings

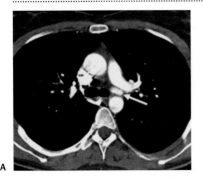
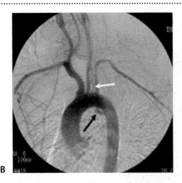
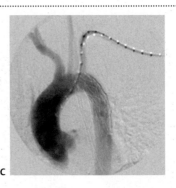

A   B   C

(A) Selected image from a contrast-enhanced computed tomographic (CT) scan of the chest at the level of the carina showing an irregular accumulation of contrast (*white arrow*) anterior to the proximal descending aorta and posterior to the left pulmonary artery, consistent with an aortic pseudoaneurysm. **(B)** Selected image from a digital subtraction arteriogram (DSA) of the aortic arch in a steep left anterior oblique (LAO) view demonstrating an irregular outward pouching of the proximal descending aorta, consistent with a pseudoaneurysm (*black arrow*). The left vertebral artery arises directly from the aortic arch as a normal variant (*white arrow*). **(C)** Selected image from a DSA of the aortic arch in a steep LAO view immediately after stent-graft placement. The leading end of the stent-graft is just distal to the origin of the left subclavian artery. A marking catheter was placed via the left brachial artery to delineate the origin of the left subclavian artery. The pseudoaneurysm is no longer demonstrated.

■ Differential Diagnosis

- *Chronic traumatic pseudoaneurysm of the proximal descending aorta:* The patient had a history of a head-on collision 20 years prior.
- *Ductus bump:* The ductus bump has smooth borders alongside the aortic wall. The lesion in the image shown has sharp angles, especially in the upper border.
- *Ulcerated atherosclerotic plaque:* This possibility is not supported by the normal appearance of all the other arteries seen.

■ Essential Facts

- The natural history of traumatic arterial injuries is poorly understood.
- Traumatic wounds of major arteries can result in serious delayed complications months or even years after the injury.
- Management is still indicated because of potentially severe complications.

✔ Pearls & ✘ Pitfalls

- ✔ Recent studies have demonstrated that endovascular repair is associated with less morbidity and mortality than is operative repair in acute blunt aortic injuries.
- ✔ Endovascular repair is replacing open repair as the treatment of choice for blunt aortic injuries in several centers.

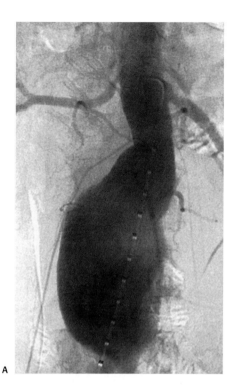

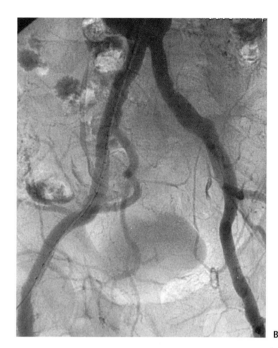

A

B

Clinical Presentation

The patient is a 67-year-old man with back pain.

■ Imaging Findings

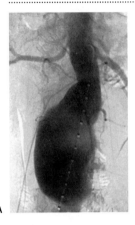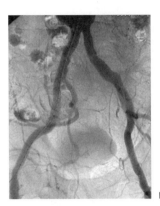

A   B

(A) Image from a nonselective digital subtraction arteriogram (DSA) of the abdominal aorta showing a large infrarenal abdominal aortic aneurysm (AAA). The distance between the lowest renal artery and the aneurysmal sac is > 15 mm. (B) Image from a DSA of the iliac arteries showing that they are patent. The iliac arteries are smooth and appear to be at least 7 mm in diameter.

■ Differential Diagnosis

• **Abdominal aortic aneurysm:** The aneurysm in this patient grew 2 cm within 1 year. Given the rate of aneurysm growth, aneurysm repair is indicated. The patient is a good candidate for endovascular repair.
• There is no differential here. The important thing is to determine whether the patient is a candidate for endovascular repair.

■ Essential Facts

• There are ~100,000 cases of AAA per year and ~15,000 related deaths per year.
• Treatment is indicated if the diameter of the aneurysm is ≥ 5 cm (with the introduction of endovascular repair, more aneurysms measuring 4.5 cm are being treated), if the aneurysmal sac grows > 0.5 cm within 6 months, or if the aneurysm is symptomatic (abdominal pain or back pain not explained by any other condition).

• The risk for rupture of an aneurysm 5 cm in diameter is 40% within 5 years.
• Approximately 60% of aneurysms can be managed with an endovascular approach (endovascular aneurysm repair, or EVAR).

✔ Pearls & ✗ Pitfalls

✔ For endovascular repair, the "healthy" infrarenal abdominal aorta must not be > 28 mm in diameter (this may change with new devices).
✔ The infrarenal neck (healthy aorta below the renal arteries) must be at least 15 mm long (this may also change with new devices).
✔ The angle between the aorta and the aneurysm should be < 60 degrees.
✔ The iliac arteries must be at least 7 mm in diameter to allow passage of the delivery system.

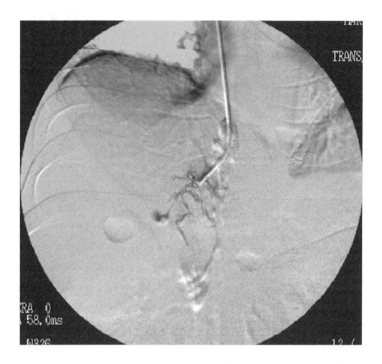

Clinical Presentation

The patient is a 29-year-old man with ascites.

■ Imaging Findings

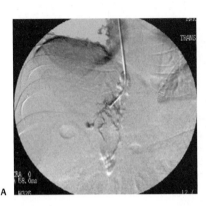 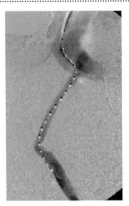

(A) Selected image from a transjugular digital subtraction hepatic venogram showing the "spider web" appearance of the hepatic veins, suggestive of hepatic venous occlusion. **(B)** Selected image from a digital subtraction direct portogram demonstrating a patent transjugular intrahepatic portosystemic shunt (TIPS).

■ Differential Diagnosis

- **Budd–Chiari syndrome:** The spider web appearance of the intraparenchymal injection of contrast is typical of Budd–Chiari syndrome.
- *Vein perforation with extravasation:* This is a possibility; however, if you look carefully at the image, the multiple tubular formations of injected contrast correspond to small, irregular vessels. A perforation or extravasation would not have this appearance.

■ Essential Facts

- Acute Budd–Chiari syndrome is a rare condition.
- It may be associated with severe, fulminant liver failure requiring emergent treatment.
- Placement of a TIPS has been proposed as one of the management options in acute Budd–Chiari syndrome associated with fulminant liver failure.

✔ Pearls & ✘ Pitfalls

- ✔ The underlying problem in Budd–Chiari syndrome is occlusion of the hepatic veins.
- ✔ Liver congestion follows, with the development of liver failure, portal hypertension, and its complications, including ascites and upper gastrointestinal bleeding.
- ✔ Liver transplantation has been the mainstay in the management of these patients.

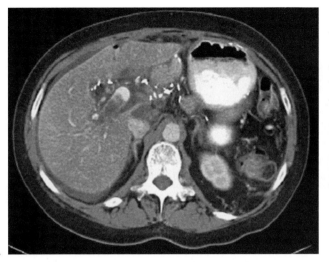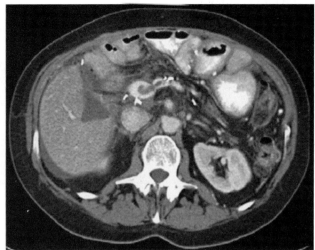

■ Clinical Presentation

The patient is a 61-year-old woman with history of pancreatic cancer.

■ Imaging Findings

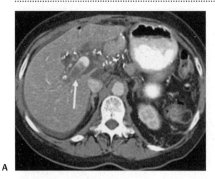
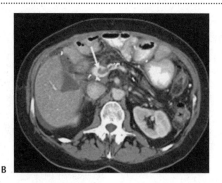
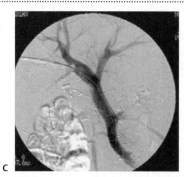

A   B   C

(A) Selected image from a contrast-enhanced computed tomographic (CT) scan of the abdomen demonstrates a large filling defect within the right branch of the main portal vein (*arrow*). **(B)** Selected image from a contrast-enhanced CT scan of the abdomen demonstrates the filling defect within the main portal vein (*arrow*). **(C)** Selected image from a digital subtraction direct portogram after percutaneous portal vein thrombectomy shows a widely patent portal vein with no residual thrombus.

■ Differential Diagnosis

- ***Acute portal vein thrombosis:*** A large filling defect within the lumen of the portal vein is surrounded by contrast. No tumor is seen. These findings are very suggestive of an acute thrombus.
- *Tumor thrombus in the portal vein:* This is a good possibility; however, it is usually associated with evidence of a mass in the liver.
- *Chronic portal vein thrombosis:* The findings do not support this possibility. Chronic portal vein thrombosis usually presents with a portal vein of decreased caliber and cavernous transformation or partial recanalization with associated periportal collaterals.

■ Essential Facts

- Spontaneous portal vein thrombosis is a rare condition.
- It may present with severe abdominal pain, liver failure, portal hypertension, and subsequent gastrointestinal bleeding.

- The therapeutic options include conservative management with systemic anticoagulation, thrombolysis via an arterial approach (usually the superior mesenteric artery), direct percutaneous transhepatic intervention in the portal vein with mechanical thrombectomy and thrombolysis, and surgical thrombectomy. The minimally invasive options are usually considered first.

✔ Pearls & ✘ Pitfalls

- ✔ Portal vein thrombosis may be related to primary coagulopathy, neoplasm, sepsis, or hypovolemia.
- ✔ Post-surgical and post-traumatic conditions may also be predisposing factors.
- ✔ Most of these cases are managed with minimally invasive techniques, with the surgical option a last resort.

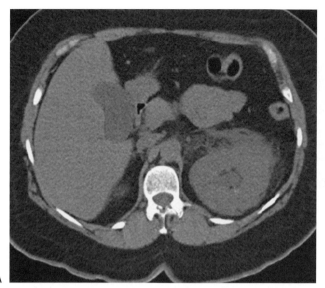

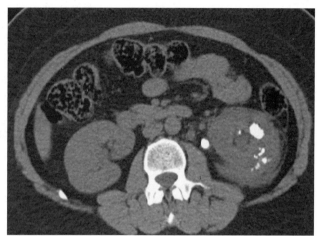

A

B

■ Clinical Presentation

The patient is a 42-year-old woman with diabetes.

■ **Imaging Findings**

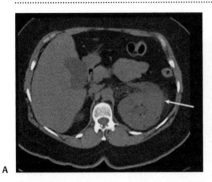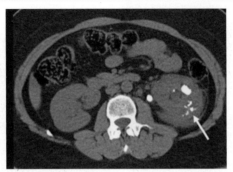

A　　　　　　　　　　　　　　　　　　　　　　　　　　B

(A) Selected image from a non–contrast-enhanced computed tomographic (CT) scan of the abdomen showing an enlarged left kidney with perirenal stranding (*arrow*). There is mild dilatation of the collecting system. (B) Selected image from a non–contrast-enhanced CT scan of the abdomen at a lower level showing multiple high-density images (*arrow*), suggestive of the presence of multiple calcifications within the collecting system. A central high-density focal image central to the left kidney is suggestive of a calcification within the proximal portion of the left ureter.

■ **Differential Diagnosis**

- *Obstructive pyelonephritis:* An enlarged kidney and perinephric stranding support this possibility. The clinical information is also useful. This patient had fever, pain, and a high white blood cell count of 19,000/mm³.
- *Pyonephrosis:* This diagnosis is difficult to make based solely on the imaging findings. A diagnosis of pyonephrosis is supported by the aspiration of purulent material after needle puncture of the collecting system.
- *Staghorn calculi:* The patient does have kidney stones, but simple stone disease does not present with enlargement and perirenal inflammation.

■ **Essential Facts**

- **Obstructive pyelonephritis is a grave condition. It is a true emergency, and treatment should not be delayed.**
- The morbidity and mortality rates of untreated obstructive pyelonephritis or pyonephrosis are very high.
- These patients require emergent decompression of the collecting system by either retrograde double-J stent placement or percutaneous nephrostomy.

✔ **Pearls & ✗ Pitfalls**

- ✔ CT is the imaging method of choice for diagnosis.
- ✔ In most centers, percutaneous drainage of the collecting system is preferred. The technical success rate is 95 to 98%.
- ✔ Twenty-five to 40% these patients will require intensive care.

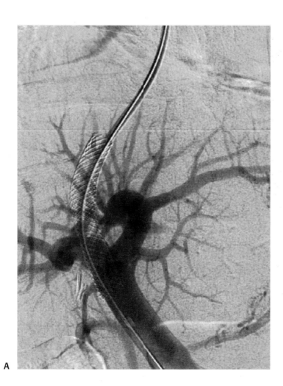

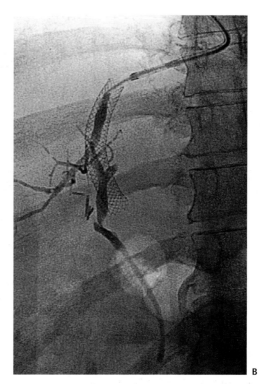

A

B

■ Clinical Presentation

Patient with an occluded transjugular intrahepatic portosystemic shunt.

■ Imaging Findings

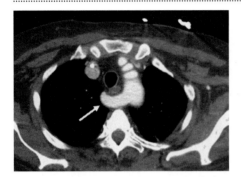

Selected image of a contrast-enhanced computed tomographic (CT) scan of the chest at the level of the aortic arch shows the origins of the right carotid artery, left carotid artery, and left subclavian artery. An additional vascular structure originates from the medial aspect of the aortic arch (*white arrow*); it is directed medially and to the right side and courses behind the esophagus. This is the last branch of the arch and is an aberrant right subclavian artery.

■ Differential Diagnosis

• ***Aberrant right subclavian artery with a left aortic arch***
• There is really no good differential diagnosis.

■ Essential Facts

• This anomaly is seen in 1 to 2% of the population.
• In this usually isolated anomaly, the right subclavian artery arises as the last branch of the aortic arch, courses from the descending aorta to the right arm, and passes behind the esophagus.

✔ Pearls & ✗ Pitfalls

✔ Aberrant right subclavian artery with a left aortic arch is usually asymptomatic (this is not a true vascular ring); however, symptoms may include dysphagia (so-called dysphagia lusoria) and dyspnea.
✔ It may be associated with a "diverticulum of Kommerell," which is a diverticulum at the origin of the anomalous vessel.

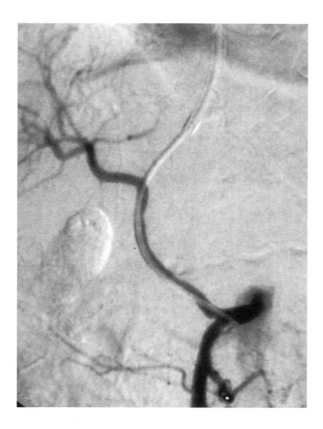

Clinical Presentation

The patient is a 46-year-old woman with primary biliary cirrhosis.

■ Imaging Findings

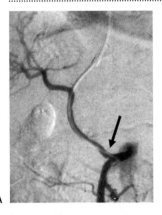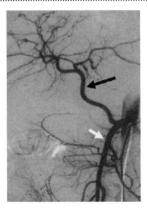

A   B

(A) Selected image from a digital subtraction arteriogram (DSA). The tip of the angiographic catheter is within the lumen of the hepatic artery (*arrow*). The image shows contrast opacification of the origin of the superior mesenteric artery and faint opacification of the abdominal aorta. The intrahepatic arterial branches are also opacified. The image is consistent with catheterization of the hepatic artery during a transjugular intrahepatic portosystemic shunt (TIPS) procedure. **(B)** Selected image from a DSA study done before the TIPS procedure in the same patient. The proper hepatic artery (*black arrow*) arises from the superior mesenteric artery (*white arrow*). This is an unusual variant seen in ~1 to 2% of the population.

■ Differential Diagnosis

• ***Hepatic arterial injury during TIPS procedure***
• *There is no differential diagnosis in this case. If the complication is not identified and the operator proceeds with the next step of the procedure, which is tract dilation and stent placement, the hemodynamic outcome may be fatal.*

■ Essential Facts

• Injury to the hepatic artery during a TIPS procedure is an unusual complication seen in < 1% of cases.
• It is a potentially fatal complication.

✔ Pearls & ✘ Pitfalls

✔ Careful evaluation of all diagnostic images obtained during a TIPS procedure is critical to identify complications.
✔ **Entry into the hepatic artery should not be confused with entry into the portal vein.**
✔ Proceeding with shunt creation in this setting would have devastating hemodynamic consequences.
✔ The recommended management of this complication is to carefully withdraw the catheter from the artery and embolize the tract.
✔ Access into the portal vein can again be attempted after the complication has been addressed.

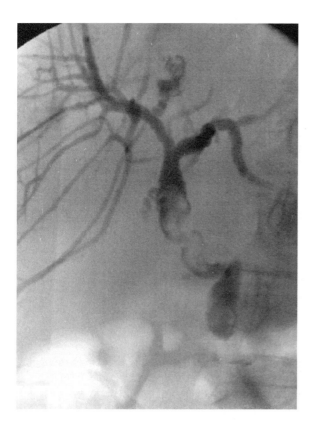

Clinical Presentation

The patient is a 64-year-old woman who has undergone a liver transplant.

■ Imaging Findings

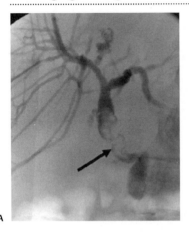
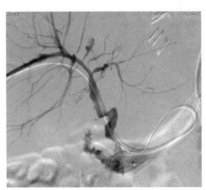

A   B

(A) Selected image from a percutaneous cholangiogram shows a large filling defect within the common bile duct (*arrow*). The filling defect conforms to the shape of the duct. No other filling defects are identified. **(B)** Digital subtraction over the wire cholangiogram via an access sheath (not shown) after the percutaneous removal of biliary casts. The common bile duct is now widely patent. No filling defects are identified.

■ Differential Diagnosis

- ***Biliary cast syndrome in a patient with a liver transplant***
- *Biliary stones:* These are usually smaller and have a better-defined shape. Biliary casts usually conform to the shape of the biliary ducts.
- *Clots within the biliary system:* This is a good possibility; the clots usually change in size and shape over time, and the patient may have clinical evidence of upper gastrointestinal bleeding.

■ Essential Facts

- Biliary cast syndrome is an unusual complication described in patients with a liver transplant.
- The etiology of cast development is not known, but it appears to be related to the accumulation of biliary sludge. Other predisposing factors include bile duct damage, ischemia, and infection.

- The present case illustrates the successful management of biliary cast syndrome with percutaneous techniques. The casts were pushed into the duodenum with a 6F Walrus balloon (Cook, Bloomington, IN).

✔ Pearls & ✘ Pitfalls

- ✔ Management is difficult; therapeutic options include endoscopic methods, surgical cast removal, and percutaneous methods. Percutaneous cast removal can be accomplished by pushing the casts into the intestine with a Fogarty-type balloon catheter. This method has been shown to be effective in some cases.

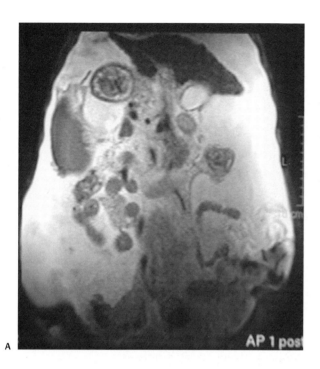

A

■ Clinical Presentation

The patient is a 67-year-old Hispanic man with liver cirrhosis and refractory ascites.

Further Work-up

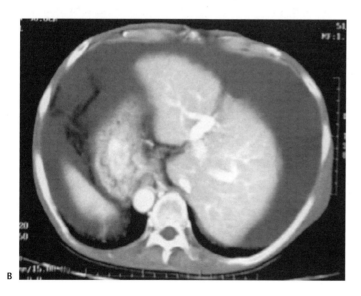

B

■ Imaging Findings

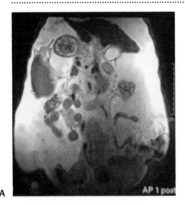

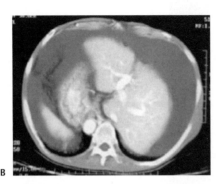

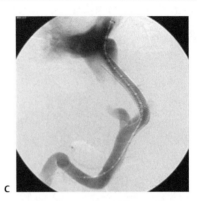

A   B   C

(A) Selected image from a magnetic resonance imaging study, coronal view, demonstrating a large amount of fluid in the abdominal cavity. The liver is small and located in the left upper quadrant. The stomach is located in the right upper quadrant, indicating complete inversion of organ distribution. (B) Selected axial image of a contrast-enhanced computed tomographic (CT) scan. This study confirms the inverse distribution of the intra-abdominal organs and the large amount of intra-abdominal fluid. Note the aorta on the right side and inferior vena cava on the left. The findings are consistent with complete situs inversus. (C) Selected image of a direct digital subtraction portogram after completion of a transjugular intrahepatic percutaneous shunt (TIPS) procedure in this patient with situs inversus.

■ Differential Diagnosis

- *TIPS procedure in a patient with situs inversus*
- There is no good differential diagnosis in this case. The most important aspect of this case is to realize that situs inversus is not a contraindication to a TIPS procedure.

■ Essential Facts

- The usual thoracic and abdominal visceral anatomy is known as situs solitus. The complete reversal of the usual anatomy is known as situs inversus totalis.

- Only two reports in the literature describe the creation of a TIPS in a patient with situs inversus.
- The procedure is carried out in the usual fashion, with the inverted anatomy kept in mind.

✔ Pearls & ✘ Pitfalls

- ✔ Careful planning of the procedure is important in cases in which the patient has a variant or unusual anatomy.
- ✔ The operator should be prepared for unexpected findings.

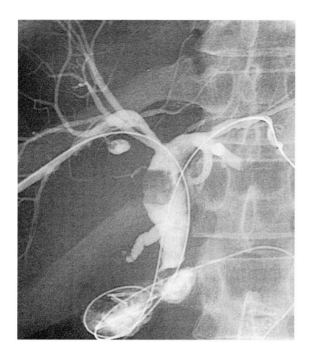

Clinical Presentation

This 57-year-old patient has undergone a liver transplant.

■ Imaging Findings

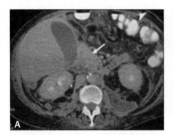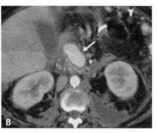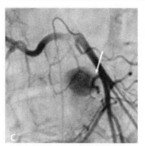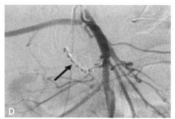

(A) Selected axial image from a delayed phase of a contrast-enhanced computed tomographic (CT) scan of the abdomen showing a soft-tissue density at the head of the pancreas (*arrow*). There is no distinct fat tissue plane between this mass and the gallbladder. **(B)** Selected axial image from a contrast-enhanced CT scan, arterial phase, showing significant contrast density within the mass. The findings are consistent with a pseudoaneurysm in the region of the pancreatic head. **(C)** Image of a selective superior mesenteric artery (SMA) injection showing that the pseudoaneurysm arises from a small branch of the SMA, most probably from the pancreaticoduodenal branches (*arrow*). Note the origin of a replaced right hepatic artery from the SMA as an incidental finding. **(D)** Image of a selective SMA injection after coiled embolization of the pseudoaneurysm shows complete obliteration of the lesion.

■ Differential Diagnosis

- ***Pseudoaneurysm of a pancreaticoduodenal artery secondary to pancreatitis***
- *Saccular aneurysm of the superior mesenteric artery:* The arteriogram shows that this lesion does not correspond to the SMA.
- *Saccular aneurysm of the gastroduodenal artery (GDA):* Involvement of the GDA in pancreatitis is relatively common, but the angiographic images show involvement of the pancreaticoduodenal arcade, not the GDA.

■ Essential Facts

- Vessel injury in acute or chronic pancreatitis is not uncommon. The most frequently affected arteries are the splenic artery (40%), gastroduodenal artery (30%), pancreaticoduodenal arteries (20%), and hepatic arteries (2%).
- If the condition is left untreated, the risk for rupture and subsequent fatal outcome is high.

- Endovascular techniques have been useful in the management of these unusual cases.
- The embolization technique is usually with coaxial catheter systems and microcoils.
- Alternatively, other agents, such as thrombin or Onyx (formerly called Embolyx, MicroTherapeutics, Irvine, CA), may be injected within the sac to occlude it. Thrombin should be administered very carefully to prevent nontarget thrombin injection, which may have catastrophic side effects.

✔ Pearls & ✘ Pitfalls

- ✔ These pseudoaneurysms should be embolized with the "sandwich" technique, in which both the distal and proximal segments of the artery feeding the pseudoaneurysm must be embolized for the procedure to be successful.
- ✔ Isolated proximal embolization is associated with recurrence of the lesion via collaterals.

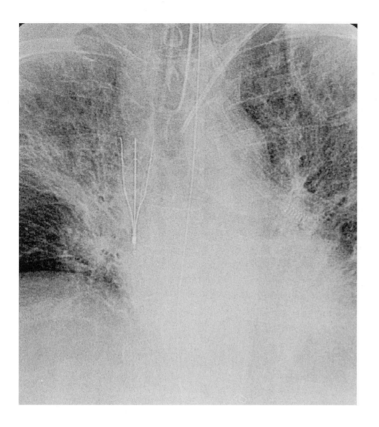

Clinical Presentation

A 57-year-old patient presents with shortness of breath.

■ Imaging Findings

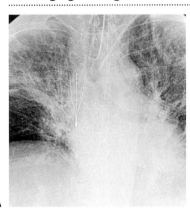 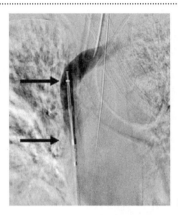

A   B

(A) Anteroposterior chest film showing large bilateral infiltrates. The patient is intubated, and the endotracheal tube is in a good position. **(B)** The tip of a left subclavian catheter is located within the left innominate vein. There is a superior vena cava (SVC) filter in a good position (*arrows*).

■ Differential Diagnosis

• **Superior vena cava filter**
• *Migrated inferior vena cava (IVC) filter:* This possibility is remote. Usually, migrated IVC filters lodge in the right atrium, the right ventricle, or rarely the pulmonary artery.

■ Essential Facts

• The placement of SVC filters was described in 1996 by Ascher and colleagues.
• The incidence of clinically significant deep vein thrombosis in the upper extremities has risen as a consequence of the increased use of indwelling central lines.
• Patients may require insertion of a central line after SVC filter placement, and this may lead to complications such as filter dislodgement or wire entrapment within the filter during attempts at placing the central line. Thus, all central line placements after SVC filter placement should be performed under fluoroscopic guidance.
• The SVC filter insertion technique includes a careful superior vena cavagram.
• Probably the easiest access is via the femoral vein. For insertion via the femoral route, a "jugular" filter should be used; thus, the filter will be deployed "upside down."
• Ideally, the filter legs should be deployed at the confluence of the innominate veins, and the filter cone should be at the most central segment of the SVC without protruding into the right atrium (Fig. B, *arrows*).

✔ Pearls & ✘ Pitfalls

✔ Reported complications include dislodgement, aortic perforation, and pneumothorax.

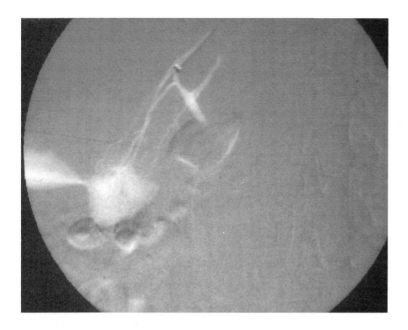

■ Clinical Presentation

The 65-year-old patient is undergoing a transjugular intrahepatic portosystemic shunt (TIPS) procedure.

■ **Imaging Findings**

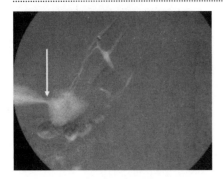

Selected image from a digital subtraction wedge hepatic venogram showing massive extravasation of contrast into the peritoneal cavity (*arrow*). This image is characteristic of capsular perforation during wedge hepatic venography.

■ **Differential Diagnosis**

• *Capsular perforation during hepatic vein wedge injection*
• There is no good differential diagnosis in this case, but this complication must be identified immediately and managed promptly.

■ **Essential Facts**

• Capsular perforation during wedge hepatic venography has been described as a fatal complication of either TIPS or transjugular liver biopsy.
• Management options are limited and include embolization of the tract, expedited completion of the TIPS procedure, and supportive measures, including correction of coagulopathy and close patient monitoring for the following 48 to 72 hours.

• The mechanism of injury may be related to the fast or forceful distribution of either contrast or carbon dioxide within the liver parenchyma along the path of least resistance to the edge of the liver, resulting in capsular perforation.
• The best approach is to prevent the complication. Authors have recommended gentle injection of 15 to 20 mL of carbon dioxide; forceful injection must be avoided.

✔ **Pearls & ✗ Pitfalls**

✔ When the complication is identified, the operator should not ignore it, and the patient should receive full supportive measures and be monitored at least 24 to 48 hours after the complication has occurred.

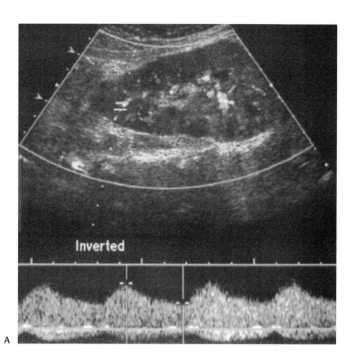

A

Clinical Presentation

The patient is a 30-year-old woman with a renal transplant.

Further Work-up

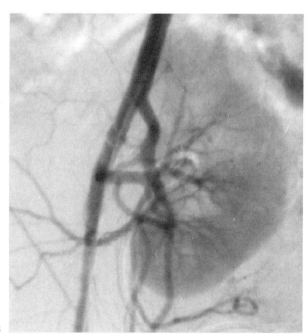

B

■ Imaging Findings

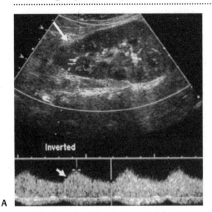 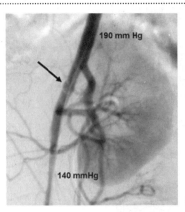

A   B

(A) Selected image from a Doppler study of the renal transplant. The interrogation is at the upper pole of the transplanted kidney in one of the arcuate branches. The waveform is "parvus et tardus" with a markedly delayed systolic upstroke (*arrow*). This finding is indicative of a significant stenosis proximal to the interrogated vessel. (B) Image from a nonselective iliac arteriogram showing a weblike lesion in the proximal portion of the external iliac artery between the origin of the internal iliac artery and the anastomosis with the transplant renal artery (*arrow*). The pressure measured at the common iliac artery is 190 mm Hg, and at the external iliac artery distal to the lesion, it is 140 mm Hg. The systolic gradient at rest is 50 mm Hg. There is no angiographic evidence of a stenosis at the anastomosis of the iliac to the renal artery or within the renal artery itself.

■ Differential Diagnosis

- ***Transplant renal artery pseudostenosis***
- *Stenosis of the transplant renal artery:* The ultrasound study supports this diagnosis; however, the answer is in the arteriogram, which shows a normal transplant renal artery.
- *Atherosclerosis of the native iliac artery:* This is unlikely in a 30-year-old patient.

■ Essential Facts

- Transplant renal artery pseudostenosis is uncommon.
- It is a lesion in the iliac artery proximal to the transplant renal artery anastomosis.
- It is most probably caused by clamp injury of the recipient iliac artery during transplant.
- This type of lesion may respond to angioplasty; however, if there is no response to angioplasty, it should be treated with a stent.

✔ Pearls & ✗ Pitfalls

- ✔ Angiographic findings in renal transplants may be difficult to interpret. Keep in mind all the diagnostic possibilities as an accurate diagnosis may save the patient's transplant.

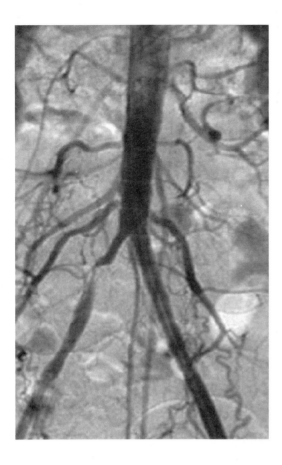

■ Clinical Presentation

The patient is a 56-year-old man with claudication of the right lower extremity.

■ Imaging Findings

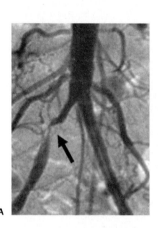 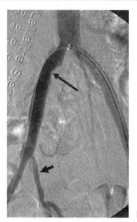

A   B

(A) Image from a digital subtraction arteriogram (DSA) of the pelvis demonstrating a severe focal stenosis of the right common iliac artery (*arrow*). Note the enlarged lumbar arteries and the lack of opacification of the right internal iliac artery. **(B)** Selected image from a DSA of the right common iliac artery after stent placement. Mild residual stenosis is seen in the proximal portion of the right common iliac artery (*arrow*). The internal iliac artery is now clearly opacified (*arrowhead*).

■ Differential Diagnosis

• ***Atherosclerotic iliac artery stenosis:*** A history of smoking is important to support this diagnosis.
• *Fibromuscular dysplasia:* This disease entity may involve the iliac arteries; however, in an older patient who is a smoker, it is not the first diagnostic option.
• *Radiation injury:* This is not a good option in a patient who has no history of previous radiation.

■ Essential Facts

• This is a category 2 lesion (eccentric stenosis < 3 cm in length) and is amenable to endovascular treatment with an expected good result.

Class 1	Focal stenosis, < 3 cm, noncalcified
Class 2	Stenosis 3–5 cm or eccentric/calcified lesions < 3 cm
Class 3	Stenosis 5–10 cm or chronic occlusions < 5 cm
Class 4	Stenoses > 10 cm, occlusions > 5 cm, extensive atherosclerotic disease bilaterally

• The advantages of primary stent placement are a high technical success rate, a shorter procedure, and minimal risk for post-intervention dissection.
• The disadvantage is the cost of the procedure.

✔ Pearls & ✘ Pitfalls

✔ The practice of primary stent placement is controversial. No prospective randomized trials demonstrating better long-term results with primary stent placement than with angioplasty have been published.

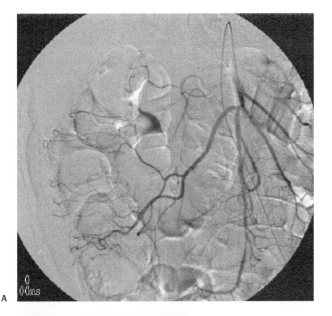
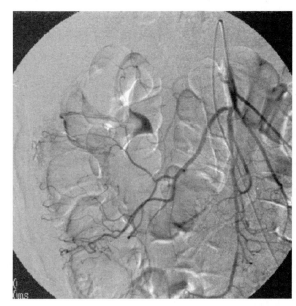

A

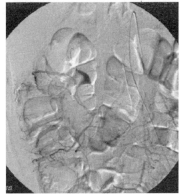

B

■ Clinical Presentation

The patient is a 62-year-old woman with gastrointestinal (GI) bleeding.

■ Imaging Findings

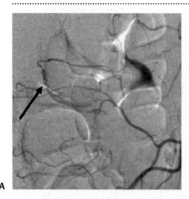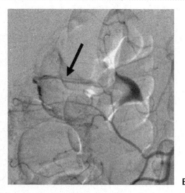

A   B

(A) Image from a selective digital subtraction arteriogram (DSA) of the superior mesenteric artery (SMA) with enlargement of the area of interest. The image shows a discrete irregularity of the vasa recta of a branch from the ileocolic artery supplying the ascending colon in close proximity to the hepatic flexure (*arrow*). All other areas seen in this figure are normal. **(B)** Image of the same area from a later phase in the arteriogram shows early opacification of a small draining vein (*arrow*).

■ Differential Diagnosis

- *Colonic angiodysplasia:* The vascular blush/irregularity and early draining vein are very suggestive of this diagnosis. There is no active GI bleeding.
- *Active bleeding in the ascending colon:* The films do not show active bleeding at the site.
- *Inflammatory lesion in the ascending colon:* There is no active bleeding, so this possibility is difficult to defend.

■ Essential Facts

- Colonic angiodysplasia is a lesion with small, dilated, thin-walled submucosal veins and capillaries.
- These are acquired lesions, usually in patients older than 60 years of age.

- The most common colonic location is the cecum, and multiple lesions are common.
- The classic angiographic appearance is that of a vascular tuft with an early draining vein.

✔ Pearls & ✘ Pitfalls

- ✔ Chances of a positive result on the angiogram increase if the patient has active bleeding during the examination (≥ 0.5 mL/min).
- ✔ A high-quality arteriogram is essential. The use of intraprocedural drugs such as glucagon, to paralyze the bowel, and papaverine, which is a vasodilator, is useful to improve image quality.

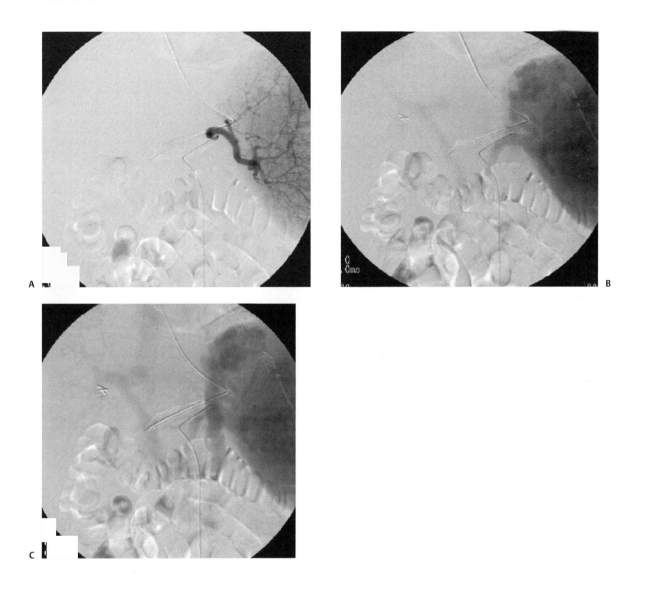

Clinical Presentation

The patient is a 64-year-old woman with a massive gastrointestinal (GI) bleed.

■ Imaging Findings

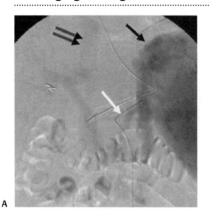
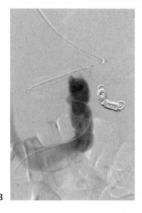
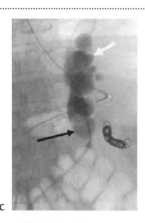

A   B   C

(A) Late phase of a selective splenic artery injection shows large gastric varices (*black arrow*) but no esophageal varices. The course of the splenic vein appears interrupted and is abnormal (*white arrow*). There is faint opacification of the inferior vena cava (*double black arrows*). **(B)** Image from a selective catheterization of the left adrenal vein. Contrast injection demonstrates large gastric varices draining into the adrenal vein. Note the coils that have been deployed in the splenic artery. **(C)** Selected image obtained during balloon-occluded retrograde embolization of the splenorenal shunt. The occlusion balloon has been selectively placed within the left adrenal vein (*black arrow*). A combination of absolute ethanol and contrast has been injected for sclerotherapy of the gastric varices (*white arrow*).

■ Differential Diagnosis

- ***Splenic vein occlusion with a large splenorenal shunt:*** The splenic vein is discontinuous, and there is late opacification of the inferior vena cava, indicating a portosystemic shunt.
- *Gastric varices:* The patient does have gastric varices, but you should be able to identify the splenic vein occlusion and the splenorenal shunt. Note that there is no reflux into esophageal varices.

■ Essential Facts

- The causes of splenic vein thrombosis include acute and chronic pancreatitis, pancreatic carcinoma, celiac and splenic artery aneurysms, and retroperitoneal fibrosis.
- Balloon-occluded retrograde embolization of gastric varices is a technique that was described in Japan by Kanagawa et al.

- It is a minimally invasive technique used to occlude gastric varices via a patent gastrorenal shunt that empties into an enlarged left adrenal vein.
- The technique requires knowledge of the anatomy of the collaterals communicating between the short gastric veins and the adrenal vein.

✔ Pearls & ✗ Pitfalls

- ✔ The presence of large gastric varices without esophageal varices is indicative of splenic vein occlusion until proven otherwise.

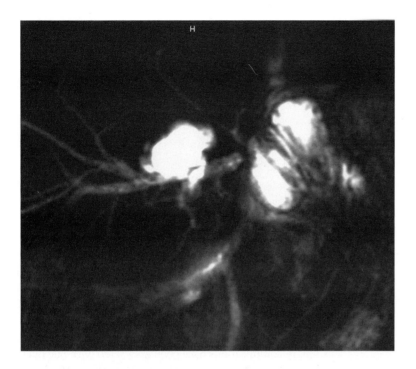

Clinical Presentation

This is a 55-year-old patient with a liver transplant.

■ Imaging Findings

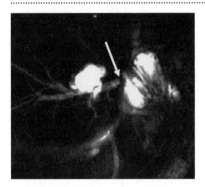

Selected image from a magnetic resonance cholangiopancreatography (MRCP) three-dimensional sequence demonstrates a large collection of bile within the liver parenchyma. There is direct communication with the biliary system. The bilioenteric anastomosis is patent, with opacification of a jejunal loop (*arrow*).

■ Differential Diagnosis

- *Bile lake; cysts in the biliary system related to biliary ischemia secondary to post-transplant hepatic artery occlusion:* Clinical information is useful.
- *Biloma:* This is usually more peripheral; it is difficult to distinguish one from the other.
- *Cholangitic abscess:* These lesions are usually peripheral and associated with the biliary system; however, they are not typically associated with ischemia.

■ Essential Facts

- The biliary tract in patients with a liver transplant is very sensitive to ischemia.
- Biliary complications occur in 15 to 20% of patients with a liver transplant and consist mainly of obstruction and leaks.
- Split liver transplants and living donor liver transplants are associated with an increased risk for biliary complications.

- Biliary complications have been associated with bile duct ischemia caused by either hepatic artery thrombosis or stenosis.
- The management of biliary complications may be difficult; the options include surgery, endoscopic management, and percutaneous techniques.
- Endoscopic management is the first line of treatment in patients with intact anatomy (patients who have a duct-to-duct anastomosis with the common bile duct draining into the second portion of the duodenum). Patients who have a bilioenteric anastomosis with a Roux-en-Y are extremely difficult to evaluate endoscopically, and percutaneous access is the first line of evaluation and treatment.

✔ Pearls & ✘ Pitfalls

- ✔ Biliary complications after a liver transplant are relatively common. Knowledge of the anatomy and type of anastomosis created is essential for correct interpretation of the images.

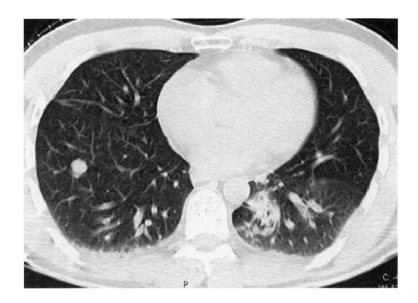

■ Clinical Presentation

The patient is a 41-year-old man with a nonproductive cough and a history of colon cancer.

■ **Imaging Findings**

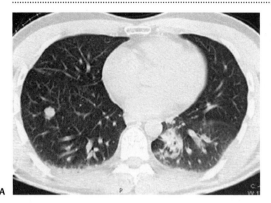 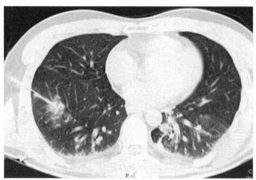

A   B

(A) Selected axial image from a computed tomographic (CT) scan of the chest demonstrates a round mass with spicules in the right lower lobe. This is highly suggestive of a metastatic lesion or primary lung carcinoma. **(B)** Selected axial image from a CT scan obtained during radio-frequency ablation (RFA) of the mass. The radio-frequency needle is seen within the mass. A discrete area of ground glass appearance surrounding the tumor is most probably related to mild hemorrhage or heat effect during the procedure.

■ **Differential Diagnosis**

- ***Metastatic lesion to the lung:*** Treatment is with lung RFA. The history is important here. The fact that the patient has history of colon cancer makes metastatic disease the first possibility.
- *Primary lung carcinoma:* This would be a very good option if patient did not have a history of previous cancer.
- *Granuloma:* No calcifications are seen, so granuloma is not a good option.
- *Pulmonary arteriovenous (a-v) malformation:* The CT does not show a feeding vessel and a draining vein, which are necessary elements to make a diagnosis of pulmonary a-v malformation.

■ **Essential Facts**

- RFA of lung tumors was first described in 2000, and its use has rapidly increased.
- RFA is minimally invasive and provides maximal preservation of normal parenchyma.
- Most procedures are performed with the patient under conscious sedation; some require general anesthesia.
- Lesions that can be treated with this method range between 1.5 and 5.2 cm in diameter.
- Pneumothorax is the most frequent complication. It occurs in ~40% of patients, with 10 to 15% requiring intervention.
- The mortality rate associated with this procedure is 0 to 5.6%.
- Most centers use contrast-enhanced CT or positron emission tomography for imaging follow-up after ablation.

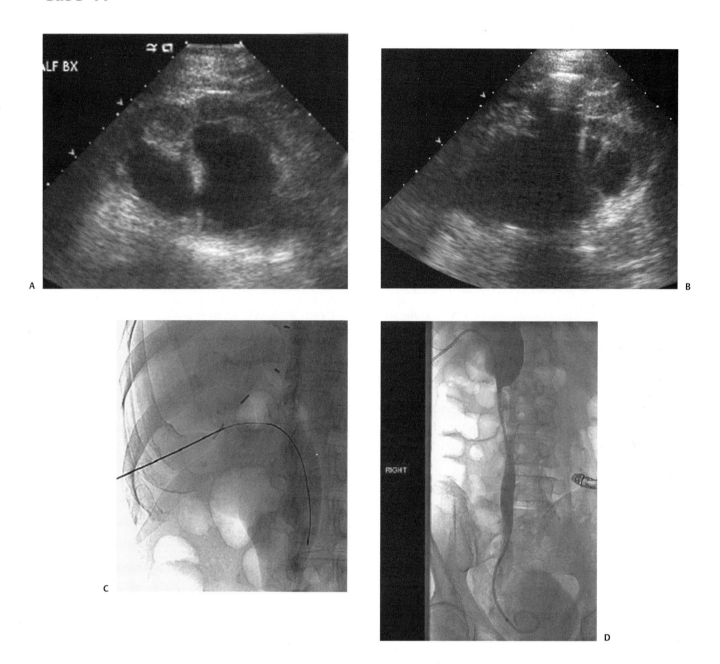

Clinical Presentation

This is a 55-year-old patient with left back pain.

■ Imaging Findings

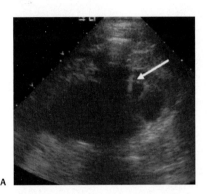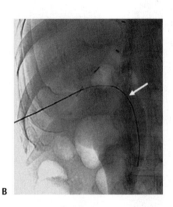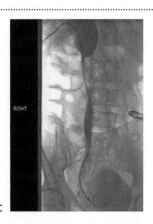

A   B   C

(A) Image obtained during ultrasound-guided percutaneous nephrostomy (PCN) tube placement. A posterior calyx of the lower pole of the kidney has been selected for access. The needle used for access is clearly demonstrated entering the calyx (*arrow*). **(B)** Spot film obtained during PCN tube placement. The needle was placed into a posterior calyx of the lower pole of the kidney under sonographic guidance. A small amount of diluted contrast has been injected through the access needle to opacify the collecting system. A wire has been advanced into the collecting system and is seen to be within the renal pelvis (*arrow*). **(C)** Spot film obtained after nephro-ureteral stent placement. The access to the collecting system seen in previous images has been used to advance a pigtail catheter into the urinary bladder.

■ Differential Diagnosis

- ***Hydronephrosis requiring PCN tube placement***
- There is no differential diagnosis for this case. The importance is to identify hydronephrosis and establish the need for percutaneous drainage.

■ Essential Facts

- The most common indication for PCN tube placement is urinary obstruction. Other indications include pyonephrosis, urinary fistulas, access for percutaneous nephrolithotomy, and hemorrhagic cystitis.
- The technique described here is the single-puncture technique. The patient is placed in the prone position. Ultrasound guidance is used for needle placement. The access of choice is a posterior calyx of the lower pole of the kidney.

Once adequate needle position is confirmed within the collecting system, a small amount of diluted contrast is injected to opacify the collecting system. The procedure is now conducted under fluoroscopic guidance. A wire is advanced into the collecting system. Tract dilation is then performed with sequentially larger dilators. Next, a drainage catheter is advanced into the renal pelvis or urinary bladder to provide drainage of the collecting system.

✔ Pearls & ✘ Pitfalls

- ✔ Avoid traversal of the pleural space (if possible avoid an intercostal approach), and avoid puncture of adjacent organs such as the liver, spleen, and colon. Be careful with the renal vascular structures.
- ✔ All patients undergoing PCN tube placement should receive a dose of prophylactic intravenous antibiotics 1 hour before the procedure.

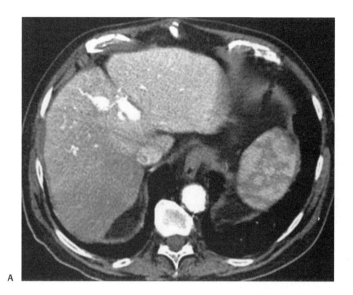

A

■ Clinical Presentation

The patient is an 80-year-old man with a liver mass and rapid deterioration of his liver function test values.

Further Work-up

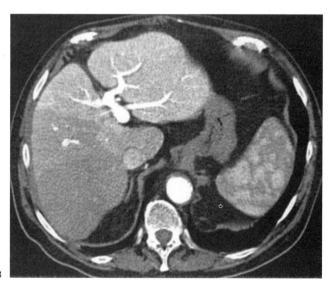

B

■ Imaging Findings

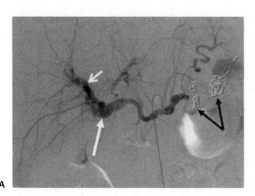 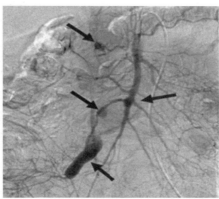

(A) Image from a selective digital subtraction arteriogram (DSA) of the celiac trunk. The hepatic artery is patent. A large fusiform aneurysm of the common hepatic artery is demonstrated (*long white arrow*), as well as multiple small fusiform aneurysms within the right hepatic artery (*short white arrow*). The splenic artery is partially occluded by multiple metallic coils (*double black arrows*). No active bleeding is demonstrated. (B) Image from a selective DSA of the superior mesenteric artery (SMA). Multiple fusiform aneurysms are identified within the branches of the SMA (*black arrows*). There is no evidence of active bleeding.

■ Differential Diagnosis

- ***Ehlers–Danlos syndrome (EDS) type 4 with multiple fusiform aneurysms in the visceral arteries***
- *Polyarteritis nodosa:* This disease process must be included in the differential. The clinical history is important.
- *Neurofibromatosis:* This disease process must be included in the differential. The clinical history is important.
- *Fibromuscular dysplasia:* This disease process must be included in the differential. The clinical history is important.

■ Essential Facts

- Vascular EDS is a rare autosomal-dominant disorder that results from a mutation of the gene encoding type 3 collagen.
- Complications are rare in childhood and appear later in life; up to 25% of cases develop before the age of 20, and 80% before the age of 40. The affected vessels are usually medium-sized arteries.
- The most common cause of death is arterial rupture. Arterial dissections are also seen in these patients.
- There is no optimal therapy for this condition. EDS type 4 usually results in premature death before age 50.

✔ Pearls & ✗ Pitfalls

- ✔ The keys to diagnosis include family history, clinical appearance, and age of the patient at presentation.

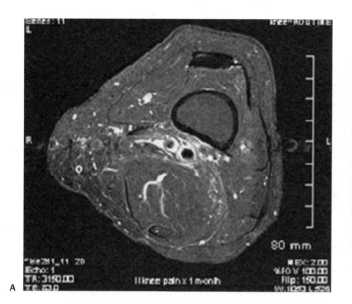 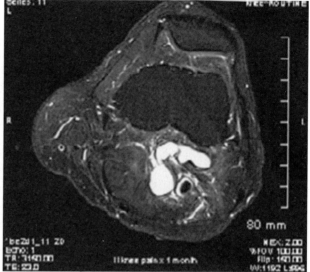

A   B

■ Clinical Presentation

The patient is a 50-year-old woman with no previous medical history.

■ Imaging Findings

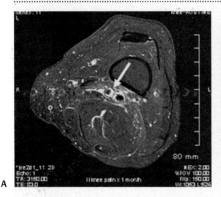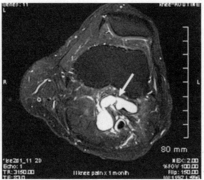

A   B

(A) Selected enhanced T1-weighted axial image of the right knee demonstrating a rim of high signal intensity surrounding the wall of the popliteal artery (*white arrow*). The popliteal vein is spared.
(B) Selected enhanced T1-weighted axial image of the right knee at a lower level demonstrating large, irregularly shaped cysts surrounding the popliteal artery and compressing its lumen (*white arrow*). The popliteal vein remains free of involvement.

■ Differential Diagnosis

- *Cystic adventitial disease of the popliteal artery:* The findings are characteristic.
- *Popliteal entrapment:* No signs of entrapment are demonstrated in this film.
- *Popliteal aneurysm:* No evidence of popliteal aneurysm is identified in the images.

■ Essential Facts

- Cystic adventitial disease is characterized by cystic degeneration of a peripheral artery.
- It was originally described as a lesion in the iliac artery; however, the popliteal artery is probably the most common site.
- This entity typically affects young to middle-aged patients with no evidence of atherosclerosis.

- Affected patients typically present with the sudden onset of calf claudication and leg pain.
- The cysts are filled with a thick mucinous gel containing varying combinations of mucoproteins, mucopolysaccharides, hyaluronic acid, and hydroxyproline.
- Treatment options include aspiration of the cyst (not recommended because of the high incidence of recurrence) and stenting of the popliteal artery (has been attempted but is usually associated with clinical failure).
- The best therapeutic option is surgical excision of the cyst with or without venous patching.

✔ Pearls & ✗ Pitfalls

- ✔ The magnetic resonance imaging appearance of cystic adventitial disease is quite characteristic, showing multiple arterial intramural cystlike masses.

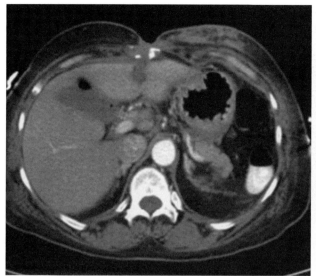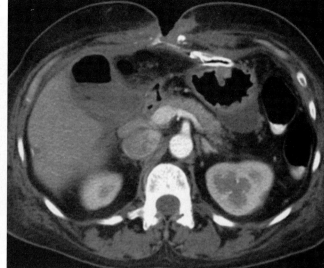

A   B

Clinical Presentation

The patient is a 55-year-old woman with severe abdominal pain and fever.

■ Imaging Findings

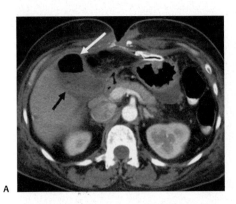
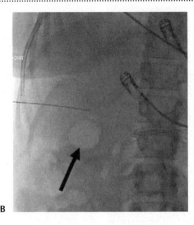
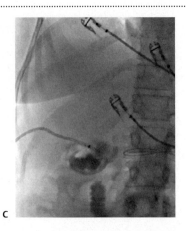

A   B   C

(A) Selected axial image from a contrast-enhanced computed tomographic (CT) scan of the abdomen at the level of the gallbladder showing thickening of the gallbladder wall (*black arrow*) and air within the gallbladder lumen (*white arrow*). **(B)** Spot film obtained during percutaneous cholecystostomy showing the puncture needle directed to the air-filled gallbladder (*arrow*). **(C)** Spot film obtained immediately after cholecystostomy tube placement showing the pigtail catheter within the gallbladder lumen. There is no extravasation of contrast.

■ Differential Diagnosis

• **Emphysematous cholecystitis (pneumocholecystitis):** The presence of air and stranding peripheral to the gallbladder are very suggestive. There is no history of previous biliary surgery to suggest abscess.
• *Abscess in the gallbladder fossa:* In the absence of a clinical history, this diagnosis is difficult to support.

■ Essential Facts

• Acute emphysematous cholecystitis is a rare entity.
• The condition is caused by gas-forming bacteria. It is more common in patients with diabetes.
• *Clostridium welchii* and *Escherichia coli* have been the most commonly isolated bacteria.

• The condition has an ischemic component but does not appear to be related to gallstones.
• The mortality rate is 15 to 20%, owing to the increased incidence of gangrene and perforation of the gallbladder wall in these patients.
• Percutaneous cholecystostomy tube placement is a noninvasive therapeutic alternative in the management of these acutely sick patients.

✔ Pearls & ✘ Pitfalls

✔ The technical success rate for percutaneous cholecystostomy tube placement is close to 100% with the combined use of sonographic and fluoroscopic guidance.
✔ Preferably, the tract should have a transhepatic course to reduce the risk for biliary peritonitis.

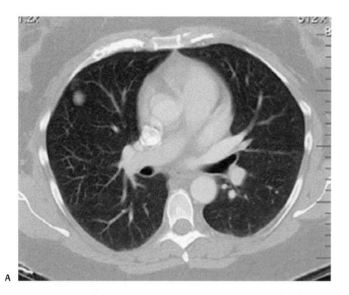
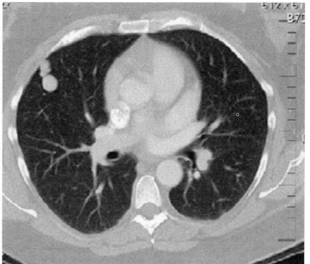

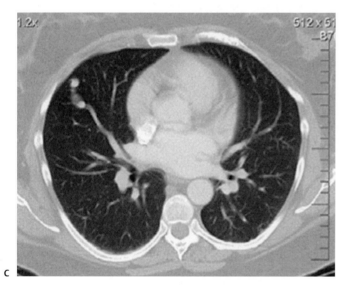

▪ Clinical Presentation

The patient is a 40-year-old woman with shortness of breath and epistaxis.

■ Imaging Findings

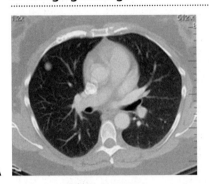 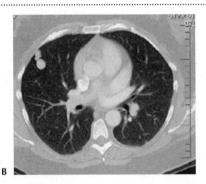 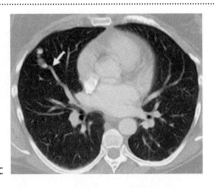

A   B   C

(A–C) Selected axial images from a contrast-enhanced computed tomographic (CT) scan of the chest demonstrating a tubular structure in the right lower lobe that enhances with the administration of contrast. There is clear demonstration of a draining vein that can be traced back to the left atrium (*arrow*, **C**).

■ Differential Diagnosis

- ***Simple pulmonary arteriovenous (a-v) malformation:*** The diagnosis is established by the presence of a feeding artery or draining vein (Fig. C).
- *Primary lung carcinoma:* This is a good possibility if only one slice is shown and has to be part of the differential.
- *Granuloma:* No calcifications are seen; this is not a good option, but you could include it in the differential.

■ Essential Facts

- Pulmonary a-v malformations are abnormal vessels connecting the pulmonary arterial circulation with the pulmonary venous circulation.
- Eighty-five percent are simple (single feeding artery/single draining vein).

- Most of these lesions are congenital; 60 to 90% of patients with a pulmonary a-v malformation have hereditary hemorrhagic telangiectasia (HHT).
- In patients with HHT, the prevalence of pulmonary a-v malformation is 15 to 35%.

✔ Pearls & ✘ Pitfalls

- ✔ The preferred management is transcatheter embolization of the malformation with coils, occluding devices, or detachable balloons.
- ✔ Do not use Gelfoam or particles for embolization as these will enter the peripheral circulation.
- ✔ If left untreated, patients are at risk for the development of neurologic problems such as stroke, transient ischemic attacks, and brain abscesses.

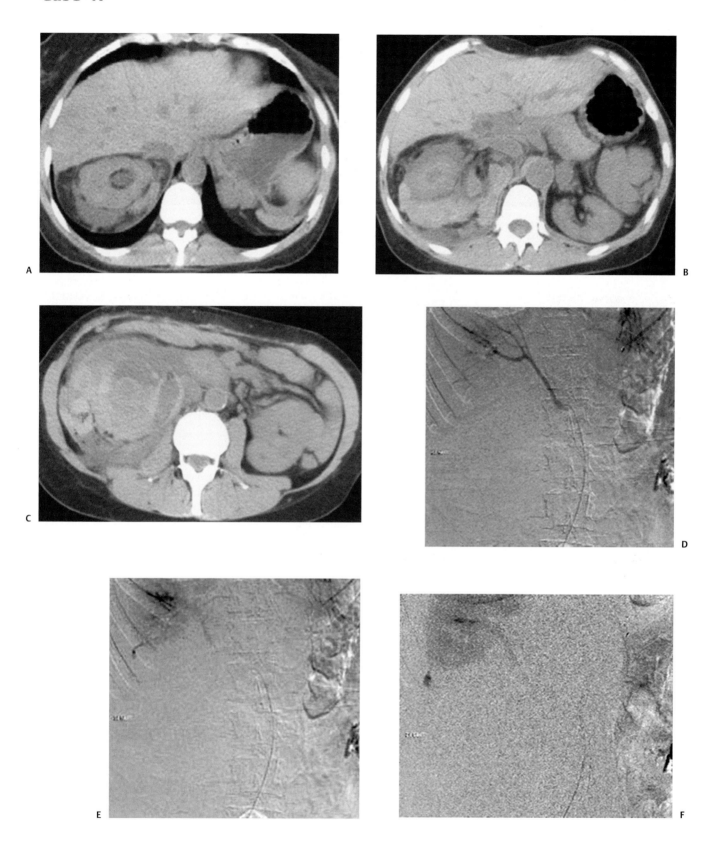

■ Clinical Presentation

The patient is a 38-year-old woman with severe abdominal pain and hematuria.

■ Imaging Findings

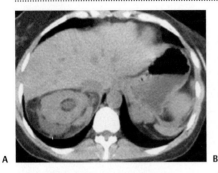
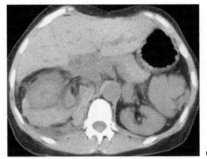
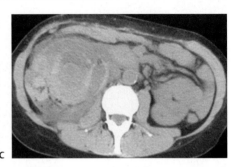

A   B   C

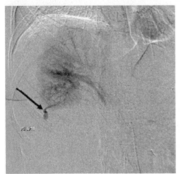
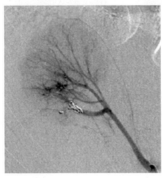

D   E

(A–C) Selected axial images from a non–contrast-enhanced computed tomographic (CT) scan of the abdomen demonstrating a large perinephric hematoma. Note the different densities seen within the large hematoma, which are suggestive of recent or even active bleeding. **(D)** Selected digital subtraction image obtained during a selective injection of the right renal artery. The arteriogram demonstrates active extravasation at the lower pole of the kidney (*arrow*). **(E)** Selected digital subtraction image obtained after superselective embolization of the segmental branch to the lower pole of the right kidney. The extravasation is no longer demonstrated.

■ Differential Diagnosis

- ***Iatrogenic injury to a renal artery after percutaneous biopsy:*** The clinical history is of great importance in a case like this. The patient was 38 years old and had just undergone a kidney biopsy.
- *Spontaneous perirenal hematoma:* This is unusual but may be seen in patients on anticoagulant therapy.
- *Renal tumor:* Not a good option in this case given the history and findings.

■ Essential Facts

- Severe back pain and tachycardia are strong clinical indicators of a complication after percutaneous biopsy. The clinician should not delay further imaging evaluation in these patients.
- Non–contrast-enhanced CT is probably the most reliable imaging method to identify a complication after percutaneous biopsy.

✔ Pearls & ✘ Pitfalls

- ✔ Arteriogram should not be delayed if there is a strong clinical suspicion of active bleeding.
- ✔ Superselective transcatheter embolization with coils or microcoils is the treatment of choice in a case of active bleeding.

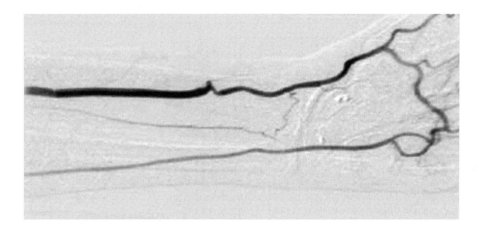

■ Clinical Presentation
....

The patient is a 65-year-old man with end-stage renal disease.

■ Imaging Findings

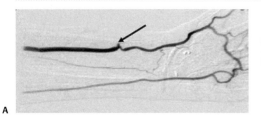
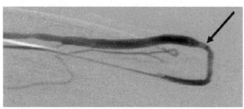

A   B

(A) Digital subtraction arteriogram (DSA) obtained with a catheter placed within the left brachial artery. The injection demonstrates a patent radial artery and ulnar artery and a complete palmar arch. A small triangular irregularity seen in the distal radial artery corresponds to the stump of a side-to-end arteriovenous (a-v) fistula between the distal radial artery and the cephalic vein (*arrow*). The a-v fistula is occluded. (B) DSA obtained after the a-v fistula had been declotted. Note that the a-v anastomosis is now widely patent (*arrow*). There is no flow into the distal radial artery, and all the flow is via the outflow vein. The fistula is now patent.

■ Differential Diagnosis

- *Occluded arteriovenous fistula:* The history is important. Previous surgery is the clue to the diagnosis.
- *Small aneurysm of the radial artery:* This is a possibility, but the history indicates the diagnosis.

■ Essential Facts

- Native a-v fistulas are the vascular access of choice for hemodialysis because their durability and patency rates are better than those of dialysis access grafts.
- Native a-v fistulas require a maturation period of ~6 weeks.
- Declotting an a-v fistula is more complex than declotting an a-v graft.

✔ Pearls & ✘ Pitfalls

- ✔ The expected technical success rate for declotting an a-v fistula ranges between 75 and 87%.
- ✔ The clinical success rate is ~80%.
- ✔ The use of thrombolytic drugs is usually necessary to open native a-v fistulas. The primary patency rates after declotting are somewhat low, in the range of 40% at 6 months and 20% at 12 months.

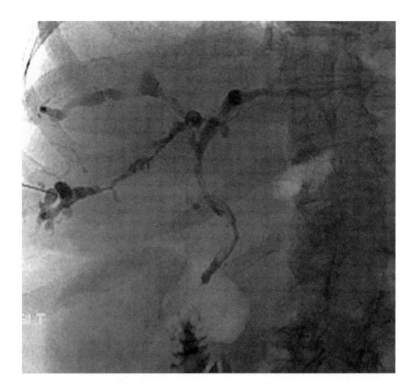

Clinical Presentation

The patient is a 73-year-old woman with jaundice.

■ Imaging Findings

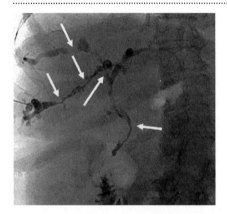

Spot film from a percutaneous cholangiogram. The biliary system shows multiple stenotic areas within the intrahepatic and extrahepatic ducts (*arrows*) alternating with areas of irregular dilation of the ducts. These findings are suggestive of areas of inflammation causing severe stenosis within the entire biliary system.

■ Differential Diagnosis

- **Primary sclerosing cholangitis (PSC):** This is high on your list. In the absence of a biopsy, it is your first possibility.
- *Cholangiocarcinoma:* PSC is associated with cholangiocarcinoma. There may be a tumor component here. It must be included in the differential.
- *Cystic disease of the biliary system:* No cysts are seen. This should be included in the differential, but it is not your best option.

■ Essential Facts

- PSC is a chronic cholestatic liver disease characterized by inflammation and fibrosis of the bile ducts. It is associated with a high risk for cholangiocarcinoma.
- Most patients present with abnormal liver function test values.

- Other symptoms include abdominal pain, jaundice, and pruritus.
- Cholangiocarcinoma is seen in 3% of these patients.

✔ Pearls & ✗ Pitfalls

- ✔ The diagnosis is based on imaging: endoscopic cholangiography, magnetic resonance cholangiography, or percutaneous cholangiography.
- ✔ Histologically, the characteristic finding is periductal fibrosis with an "onion skin" pattern resulting in ductopenia.
- ✔ PSC is a disease of unknown etiology. The best treatment option is a liver transplant.

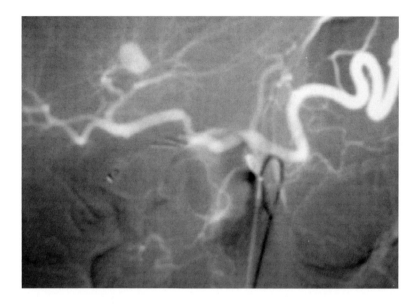

Clinical Presentation

The patient is a 64-year-old man with upper gastrointestinal bleeding.

■ Imaging Findings

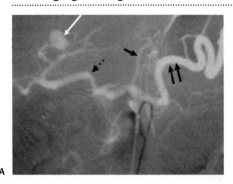 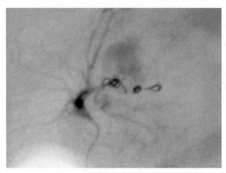

A   B

(A) Selected image from a selective injection of the celiac trunk. A large, rounded area of extravasation of contrast arises from an anterior branch of the left hepatic artery (*white arrow*). The main branches of the celiac trunk are patent: the splenic artery (*double black arrows*) and left gastric artery (*short black arrow*). The hepatic artery anastomosis is patent (*broken arrow*). **(B)** Selected image from an arteriogram after coil embolization. The pseudoaneurysm is no longer identified.

■ Differential Diagnosis

- **Hepatic artery pseudoaneurysm:** The history is important in this case. Iatrogenic trauma, such as from a previous biopsy or drainage procedure, is important. You should also consider the possibility of previous trauma.
- *Saccular aneurysm of the hepatic artery:* This is rare in the absence of a systemic vascular disease, such as Ehlers–Danlos syndrome type 4.
- *Arterioportal fistula:* No opacification of the portal vein is demonstrated.

■ Essential Facts

- Pseudoaneurysms of the hepatic artery are uncommon lesions that are usually related to penetrating injury to the liver (stab wounds, biopsies, percutaneous cholangiography, and placement of biliary drainage catheters). The clinical presentation may include massive hemobilia.

- Therapeutic options include superselective embolization or, if feasible, stent-graft placement.
- A few case reports describe successful management of these lesions with direct injection of thrombin (under computed tomographic or ultrasound guidance).

✔ Pearls & ✗ Pitfalls

✔ Endoscopic evaluation and management of patients who have a liver transplant with a bilioenteric anastomosis and the creation of a Roux-en-Y limb is limited because of the technical difficulty encountered in manipulating the endoscopy tube to the biliary anastomosis through the Roux-en-Y limb. These patients are better managed with endovascular or percutaneous techniques.

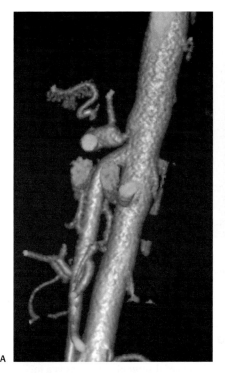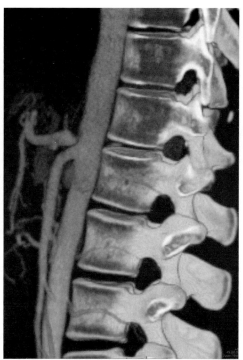

A   B

■ Clinical Presentation

An 18-year-old patient presents with post-prandial abdominal pain and a 23-pound weight loss.

Further Work-up

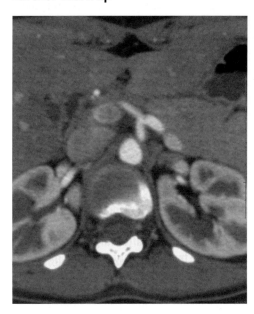

C

■ Imaging Findings

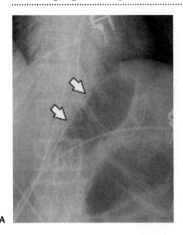
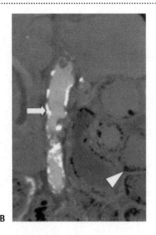
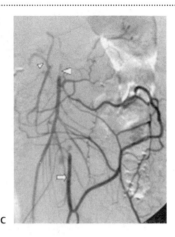

A   B   C

(A) Radiograph shows dilated loops of bowel and possible pneumatosis (*arrows*). **(B)** Contrast-enhanced computed tomography (CT) shows pneumatosis (*arrowhead*) and aortic calcifications (*arrow*). **(C)** Inferior mesenteric artery (IMA: *arrow*) angiogram shows superior mesenteric artery (SMA: *large arrowhead*) stenosis and reconstitution via the marginal artery from the IMA; the celiac artery is presumed stenotic because its branches are reconstituted via pancreaticoduodenal arteries supplied by the SMA (proper hepatic artery: *small arrowhead*).

■ Differential Diagnosis

- **Mesenteric ischemia (MI) with superior mesenteric artery and celiac artery obstruction:** The only diagnosis for all the imaging findings and the clinical presentation; the radiographic findings are nonspecific (bowel obstruction, infection, inflammation, ischemia, and ileus).

■ Essential Facts

- MI can have a variety of causes, including atherosclerosis, thrombosis, retroperitoneal fibrosis, median arcuate ligament syndrome, fibromuscular dysplasia, and Takayasu's arteritis.
- MI is typically symptomatic if the obstruction involves at least two primary mesenteric arteries.
- Mesenteric angiography in acute cases may show abrupt cutoff and thrombus and, in chronic cases, supply to obstructed arteries by collaterals from unobstructed arteries.
  - Celiac artery obstruction: collateral supply to celiac branches from the SMA via the pancreaticoduodenal arcade or arc of Buehler.
  - SMA obstruction: collateral supply to the SMA branches from the celiac artery via the pancreaticoduodenal arcade or arc of Buehler; collateral supply from the IMA via the marginal artery or arc of Riolan.
  - IMA obstruction: collateral supply to the IMA branches from the SMA via the left colic and marginal arteries or arc of Riolan; collateral supply from the internal iliac artery via retrograde flow in the superior rectal artery.

■ Other Imaging Findings

- Contrast-enhanced CT with CT angiography is usually the first step in the diagnosis of MI to establish a treatment plan. Look for bowel dilatation, bowel wall thickening, pneumatosis, arterial stenosis/thrombosis/occlusion, and enlarged collateral arteries.

✔ Pearls & ✘ Pitfalls

- ✔ Most patients with peritoneal signs and pneumatosis undergo emergent laparotomy. This patient underwent preliminary arteriography to plan the surgical resection, given the extent of atherosclerotic disease.
- ✔ Mesenteric artery stenting may be used for chronic fixed obstruction associated with atherosclerosis.
- ✔ Balloon-expandable stents are placed because the lesions are usually ostial (like renal stenosis).
- ✘ Mesenteric artery thrombolysis has been described for acute thromboembolism, but surgery replaces this treatment in most cases because of the rapid (< 12 hour) progression to ischemic bowel.
- ✘ Revascularization of nonviable bowel is contraindicated. Cases involving pneumatosis and portal venous gas typically require surgical resection combined with aortomesenteric bypass.

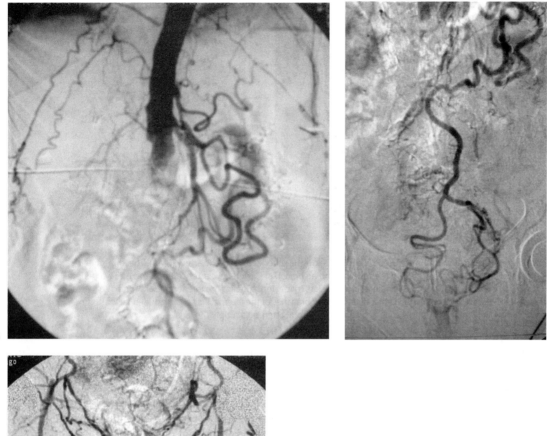

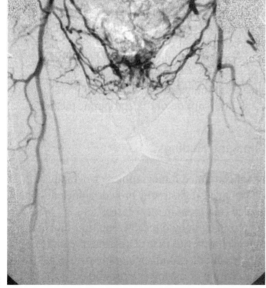

■ Clinical Presentation

A 60-year-old woman presents with buttock claudication. Pulses in the common femoral artery are not palpable.

■ Imaging Findings

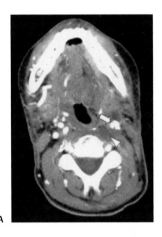
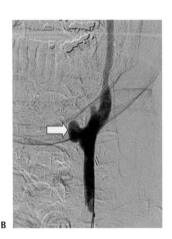
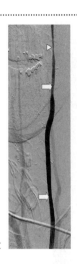

A   B   C

(A) Contrast-enhanced computed tomographic (CT) scan of the neck 3 days before carotid rupture shows an irregularly marginated left carotid artery (*arrow*) passing through necrotic neck tumor (*arrowhead*). **(B)** Conventional angiogram in the frontal projection shows pseudoaneurysm (*arrow*) of the common carotid artery within the neck tumor. **(C)** Repeat angiogram after placement of a covered stent (*arrows*) shows successful exclusion of pseudoaneurysm. Vasospasm is noted above the stent (*arrowhead*).

■ Differential Diagnosis

- ***Carotid blowout syndrome:*** Indicated by bleeding, pseudoaneurysm, and an associated head and neck tumor.

■ Essential Facts

- Defined as bleeding from the carotid artery caused by direct invasion from an adjacent necrotic neck tumor, radiation treatment, and/or surgical treatment. Less commonly, pseudoaneurysms may be caused by trauma.
- Minor bleeding may precede massive, life-threatening hemorrhage.
- Carotid artery embolization with coils and detachable balloons was formerly the only method of endovascular treatment.
- Placement of a covered stent has become a first-line treatment option.
- Surgical treatment is carotid artery ligation, which carries a high risk for stroke. Poor wound healing secondary to irradiation of tissue and poor nutritional health makes these patients poor surgical candidates.

■ Other Imaging Findings

- For minor bleeding and an appropriate clinical history, obtain an infused CT scan to make a diagnosis and plan treatment.
- For massive bleeding and an appropriate clinical history, angiography is often a first-line option for both diagnosis and treatment.
- Typical findings include pseudoaneurysm and extravasation.

✔ Pearls & ✗ Pitfalls

- ✔ Pre-procedural care may require external wound packing, and for severe bleeding, packing of the throat with concurrent tracheostomy.
- ✔ Success rates > 90% have been reported.
- ✔ The long-term durability of stents for carotid blowout syndrome has not been established.
- ✗ The risks of endovascular treatment include stent-related infection, rupture, recurrent bleeding after progression of disease, endoleak, and stroke.

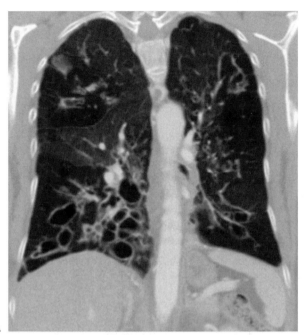

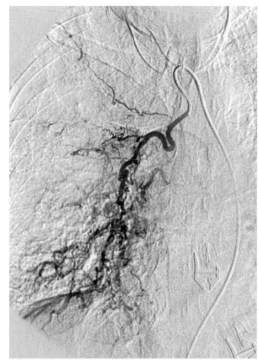

A   B

■ **Clinical Presentation**

....

A 55-year-old patient presents with hemoptysis. The rate of bleeding is estimated to be 350 mL over the past 24 hours.

Imaging Findings

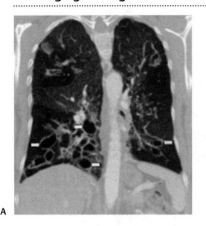
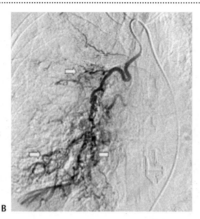

(A) Coronal contrast-enhanced computed tomographic (CT) scan shows bilateral cystic bronchiectasis (*arrows*). **(B)** Right bronchial arteriogram shows increased vascularity (*arrows*) but no active extravasation (Simmons 1 catheter).

Differential Diagnosis

- ***Cystic bronchiectasis causing massive hemoptysis:*** The only diagnostic consideration.

Essential Facts

- Massive hemoptysis (> 300 mL/d) carries a high risk for death by asphyxiation. Sources include the bronchial (90%), pulmonary (5%), and systemic arteries (5%).
- Causes include tuberculosis, fungal and bacterial infections, chronic bronchitis, sarcoidosis, cystic fibrosis, bronchogenic carcinoma, bronchial adenoma, and bronchial artery aneurysms.
- Bronchial artery embolization is the definitive treatment in most cases (surgery is indicated for neoplasms and refractory cases).
- Nonpulmonary sources include the bronchial arteries, intercostal bronchial trunks, aberrant bronchial arteries, and nonbronchial systemic arteries.
- Common variations are two left bronchial arteries with one right intercostal bronchial trunk (40%) and one left bronchial artery with one right intercostal bronchial trunk (21%).
- Aberrant bronchial arteries run parallel to the bronchi but may arise from atypical sites such as the aortic arch (most common), internal mammary arteries, subclavian artery, and costovertebral trunk.
- The nonbronchial systemic arterial supply does not run parallel to the bronchi (often seen in patients with extensive parenchymal disease).

Other Imaging Findings

- Radiography is used to diagnose (50%) and localize the abnormality for embolization or surgery.
- Bronchoscopy may localize bleeding or identify a small neoplastic bronchial lesion, but bleeding can obscure visualization.

- Multidetector CT provides high-resolution images to detect small bronchial neoplasms and interstitial lung disease. Unlike bronchoscopy, CT can evaluate the bronchi despite active bleeding.

✔ Pearls & ✘ Pitfalls

- ✔ Bronchial angiography is performed with the intent to embolize. Findings include tortuous, enlarged bronchial arteries and hypervascularity, typically without active extravasation. Bronchial arteries arise near left the main bronchus in 94% of cases (T5–T6).
- ✔ Early recurrence should prompt another search for aberrant bronchial or systemic arterial feeders.
- ✔ Particles > 325 μm (stop in pulmonary capillary bed) are used—polyvinyl alcohol or tris-acryl microspheres.
- ✔ Gelfoam particles are typically not used because of the risk for recanalization and early recurrence, and coils are avoided except for aneurysms and arteriovenous malformations (block bronchial artery embolization when symptoms recur).
- ✔ Success rates are 90% for acute hemoptysis and 65% for long-term resolution (repeat bronchial arterial embolization common).
- ✘ Complications of bronchial arterial embolization include chest pain, dysphagia, dissection, tissue necrosis (lung, bronchi, and esophagus), transient cortical blindness, and paralysis due to spinal artery embolization or injury.
- ✘ "Hairpin-shaped" anterior medullary arteries are a contraindication (arise from intercostal bronchial trunk in 10% of cases).
- ✘ The artery of Adamkewicz should not be probed (T9–T12 level in 75% of cases).

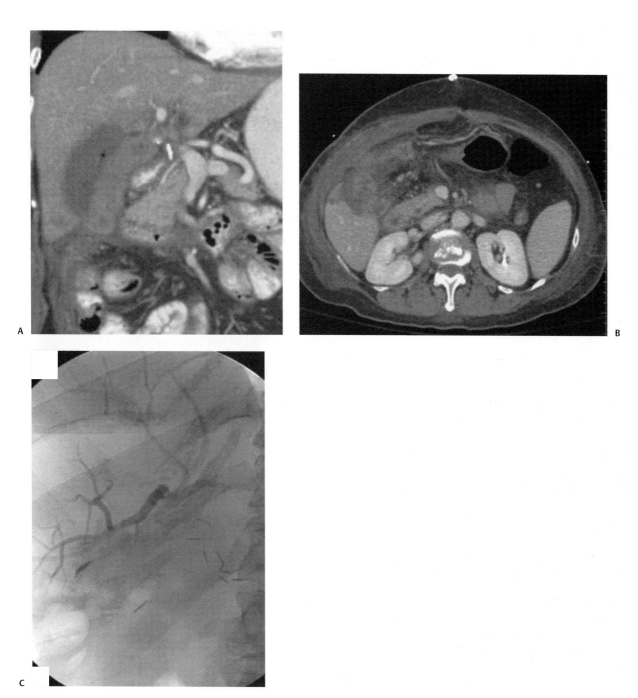

A

B

C

Clinical Presentation

A 61-year-old man presents with biliary obstruction after Roux-en-Y biliary reconstruction for cholangiocarcinoma.

■ **Imaging Findings**

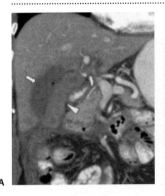
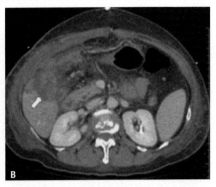
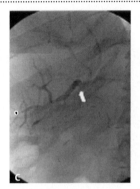
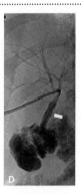

A

B

C

D

(A,B) Contrast-enhanced computed tomographic (CT) scan shows a soft-tissue mass (*arrow*) adjacent to the Roux limb (*arrowhead*). **(C)** Percutaneous cholangiogram shows central biliary obstruction (*arrow*). A biliary drain was placed for 3 days to decompress the bile ducts before stent placement. **(D)** Successful placement of stent (*arrow*) across the extrahepatic duct.

■ **Differential Diagnosis**

- **Malignant biliary obstruction:** The most likely diagnosis in the setting of a history of cholangiocarcinoma and a recurrent soft-tissue mass.
- *Abscess:* A possibility if the clinical presentation is fever and leukocytosis, but this entity is less likely to cause biliary obstruction.
- *Benign stricture of the biliary–enteric anastomosis after Roux-en-Y reconstruction:* Can cause obstruction that is not treated with permanent metallic stents, but the mass adjacent to the Roux-en-Y reconstruction makes this diagnosis unlikely.

■ **Essential Facts**

- Permanent metal stents are a standard palliative treatment for biliary obstruction resulting from incurable malignancy, including pancreatic carcinoma, cholangiocarcinoma, lymphoma, and metastasis.
- The goal is for the metallic biliary stent to remain patent beyond the life expectancy of the patient.
- Temporary plastic stents are less effective and typically not used for incurable malignancy.
- Stents may be placed via the endoscopic approach or the percutaneous transhepatic approach.

■ **Other Imaging Findings**

- Ultrasound provides an adequate evaluation of hepatic, biliary, and pancreatic tumors, but an inadequate evaluation of duodenal tumors for concurrent duodenal stent placement.
- Contrast-enhanced CT helps to plan the route of percutaneous access through the liver to avoid traversing tumors.
- Magnetic resonance cholangiopancreatography provides excellent three-dimensional imaging of the biliary tree, pancreatic duct, and duodenum for planning stent placement.

✔ **Pearls & ✗ Pitfalls**

- ✔ The endoscopic approach decreases the risk for bleeding but is not always successful. In patients with a Roux-en-Y reconstruction, as in this case, the endoscopic approach is usually not possible, and the percutaneous approach becomes the first-line option for evaluation and treatment.
- ✔ The percutaneous approach is reserved for cases with preexisting external biliary drains and cases in which the endoscopic approach has failed or is unlikely to be successful.
- ✔ Preliminary placement of an internal–external biliary drainage catheter is advisable 2 to 3 days before stent placement in patients with sepsis to decompress the biliary tree and prevent exacerbation of the sepsis.
- ✔ The mean duration of stent patency is 73 to 288 days; the mean patient survival is 194 to 214 days.
- ✔ The patency rates are better for covered stent-grafts than for bare stents, but covered stent-grafts carry an increased risk for acute cholecystitis and pancreatitis.
- ✗ Major complications (2%) of percutaneous biliary stenting include sepsis, bleeding, and death.
- ✗ Minor complications (30%) include self-limited bleeding and fever.
- ✗ Delayed complications (16%) include stent occlusion, stent migration, pancreatitis, and acute cholecystitis.
- ✗ In patients with benign lesions or focal malignancies, stent placement may interfere with surgical options. Surgical options should be considered before a metal stent is placed.

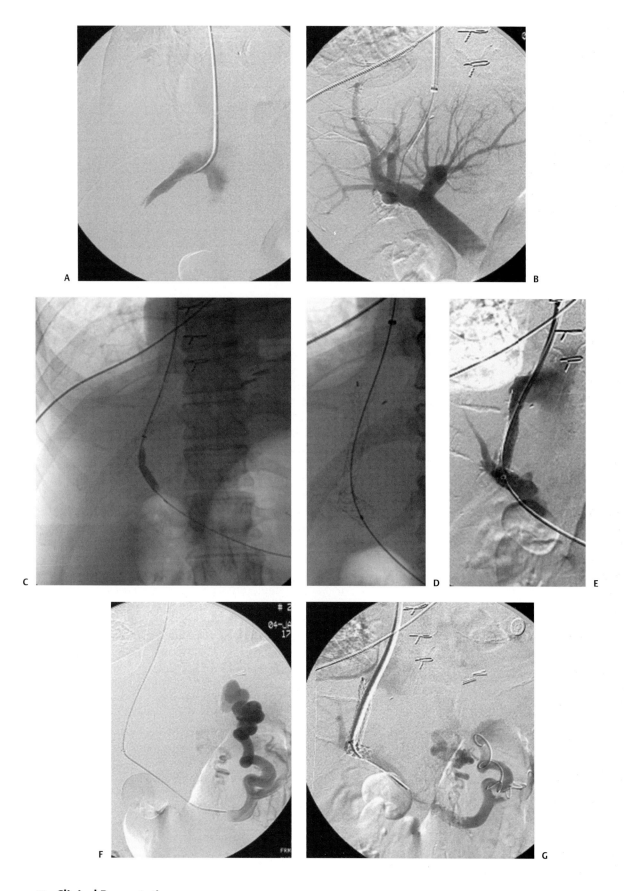

Clinical Presentation

The patient is a 56-year-old man with cirrhosis and bleeding gastroesophageal varices who is in the intensive care unit.

■ Imaging Findings

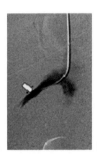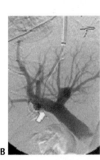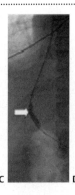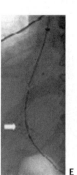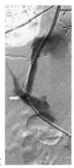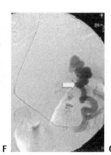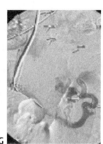

A   B   C   D   E   F   G

(A) Right hepatic (*arrow*) venogram—wedged (portal) pressure can be measured at this time. **(B)** Portal venous puncture and cannulation (*arrow*) at least 1 cm above the portal bifurcation, optimally. **(C)** Tract dilation with an 8-mm-diameter balloon (*arrow*). **(D)** Deployment of a covered stent (Viatorr stent: *arrow*). **(E)** Follow-up venogram (*arrow*); dilate stent if narrow. **(F)** Variceal venography: persistent antegrade flow despite a transjugular intrahepatic portosystemic shunt (TIPS: *arrow*). **(G)** Venography after coil (*arrow*) embolization.

■ Differential Diagnosis

• **_Transjugular intrahepatic portosystemic shunt and variceal embolization_**

■ Imaging Findings

• Indications
  • Variceal bleeding after failed medical management
  • Refractory ascites secondary to portal hypertension
  • Refractory hepatic hydrothorax
  • Hepatorenal syndrome
  • Portal gastropathy
  • Budd–Chiari syndrome
  • Veno-occlusive disease
• Contraindications (absolute)
  • Right-sided heart failure
  • Primary pulmonary hypertension
  • Polycystic liver disease
  • Severe hepatic failure
• Contraindications (relative)
  • Biliary obstruction
  • Portal vein obstruction
  • Severe encephalopathy
  • Liver or systemic infection

✔ Pearls & ✗ Pitfalls

✔ Octreotide and beta-blockers are administered for varices, diuretics and serial percutaneous drainage for ascites, hepatic hydrothorax.
✔ Endoscopy distinguishes arterial from portal bleeding and facilitates concurrent sclerotherapy.
✔ Contrast-enhanced computed tomography (CT) or Doppler ultrasound shows patency of the portal vein and demonstrates ascites, cystic liver disease, Budd–Chiari syndrome.
✔ The liver is biopsied for veno-occlusive disease; the portosystemic gradient is measured from the jugular approach.
✔ TIPS after failed endoscopic therapy arrests bleeding in nearly all cases if the portosystemic gradient is reduced to < 12 mm Hg.
✔ Model of end-stage liver disease (MELD) score < 25 predicts lower mortality risk of TIPS placement (based on serum creatinine and serum bilirubin levels, international normalized ratio, and cause of cirrhosis).
✔ Embolization of persistent varices after TIPS creation is controversial but may help control bleeding.
✔ Ultrasound should be used to confirm TIPS patency at 2 weeks, 3 months, and then every 6 months.
✔ Normal TIPS velocity is 1 m/s; increase or decrease may indicate stenosis.
✔ Surgical shunt (distal splenorenal or mesocaval) for varices is indicated if a TIPS cannot be placed.
✗ Complications:
  • Periprocedural mortality rate, 2%; 30-day mortality rate, 3 to 15%
  • Cardiac arrhythmia, heart block
  • Capsule laceration resulting from wedged hepatic venography
  • TIPS-to-bile duct fistula (bare stents)
  • Hepatic artery injury (bleeding or infarct)
  • Portal injury (bleeding or thrombosis)
  • Inferior vena cava (IVC) laceration
  • Capsule puncture (rarely significant)
  • Shunt thrombosis resulting from incomplete extension to IVC, kinking, pseudointimal hyperplasia (bare stents)
  • Hemolysis (associated with Wallstents [Boston Scientific, Natick, MA])
  • Hepatic failure, 3 to 7%
  • Hepatic encephalopathy, 10 to 20% (95% treatable)

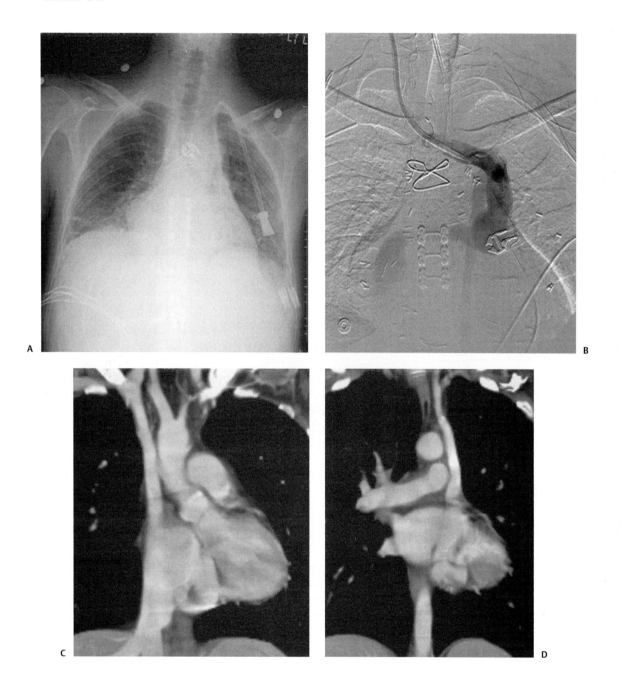

A

B

C

D

■ Clinical Presentation

A 41-year-old man presents for placement of a central line for dialysis.

■ Imaging Findings

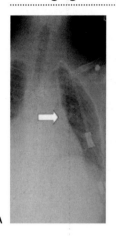 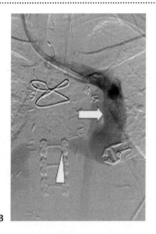 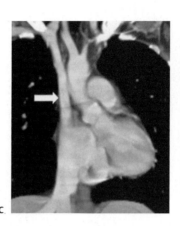 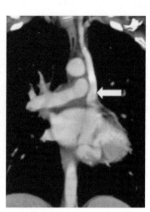

(A) Frontal radiograph shows central line along the left mediastinum (*arrow*). The line was not functioning. **(B)** Venogram from a new right jugular line shows a left-sided superior vena cava (SVC: *arrow*) with anomalous drainage into the coronary sinus (*arrowhead*). **(C)** Coronal reformatted contrast-enhanced computed tomographic (CT) scan shows patent right SVC (*arrow*). **(D)** More posterior slice shows persistent left SVC (*arrow*).

■ Differential Diagnosis

- **Persistent left superior vena cava (PLSVC):** Indicated by jugular venous drainage to a large, left mediastinal vein that ultimately drains into the right atrium. The remainder of this differential refers to the radiographic finding of a central line projecting over the left mediastinum.
- *Arterial catheterization:* Should be mentioned in all cases in which a central line courses along the left mediastinum because this complication carries a risk for hemorrhage or distal thromboembolism.
- *Enlarged mediastinal vein:* A possibility for a left mediastinal catheter but is typically associated with central venous obstruction, not present in this case.

■ Essential Facts

- PLSVC is the most common thoracic venous anomaly and presents in children or adults, depending on the venous drainage and the presence of any associated congenital heart defects.
- The cause is persistence of the embryologic left superior cardinal vein.
- The most common form (usually asymptomatic) is central venous drainage to the right atrium via the left coronary sinus.
- In a less common form (often symptomatic), alternative drainage to the left atrium occurs either directly or through an anomalous coronary sinus. Reported associated vascular and cardiac defects include absent left brachiocephalic vein, absent or anomalous right SVC, absent coronary sinus, atrial septal defect, and tetralogy of Fallot. Right-to-left shunting can result in brain abscess or stroke from paradoxical venous thromboembolus.

■ Other Imaging Findings

- Brain CT or magnetic resonance imaging (MRI) may show brain abscess or stroke from paradoxical venous thromboembolus.
- Cardiac CT or MRI may show the venous and cardiac anomalies previously listed.
- Chest radiography may show the shunt vascularity and cardiac enlargement of atrial septal defect or the boot-shaped heart of tetralogy of Fallot.

✔ Pearls & ✘ Pitfalls

- ✔ If you encounter PLSVC in a child, look for associated cardiac anomalies to explain the early clinical presentation.
- ✔ If you encounter a patient with a central line coursing along the left side of the chest, consider PLSVC, inadvertent arterial catheterization, an enlarged mediastinal collateral vein (e.g., superiormost intercostal) resulting from chronic obstruction of the left brachiocephalic vein, or inadvertent extraluminal access.
- ✘ In the less common form (drainage to the left atrium), thromboembolism from a central catheter or air from an intravenous or central catheter can result in cerebral, cardiac, or systemic embolization.
- ✘ If you encounter a patient with paradoxical thromboembolism, do not miss alternative causes, such as right-to-left cardiac shunts.

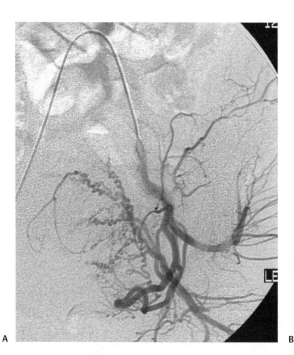

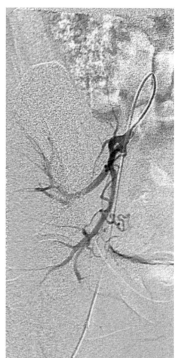

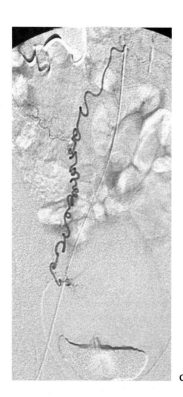

A   B   C

■ Clinical Presentation

A 46-year-old woman presents with pelvic pain and menorrhagia.

■ Imaging Findings

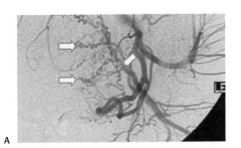
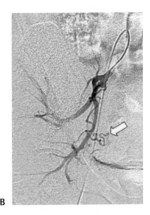
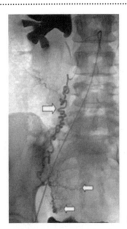

(A) Left internal iliac arteriogram shows large branches of the uterine artery (UA) supplying fibroids (*arrows*). The UA was embolized with polyvinyl alcohol particles. **(B)** Right internal iliac arteriogram shows a very small UA supplying fibroids (*arrow*). **(C)** Selected right ovarian (*large arrow*) arteriogram shows direct supply to the uterus (*small arrows*). The uterine branches were embolized.

■ Differential Diagnosis

- *Uterine artery embolization (UAE) with ovarian artery supply*

■ Essential Facts

- Fibroids affect 30 to 40% of women older than 35 years of age.
- Symptoms (in 25%) consist of metromenorrhagia (severe bleeding, anemia) or are bulk-related (urinary frequency, physical discomfort, constipation).
- Types include subserosal (least likely to cause symptoms or respond to UAE), intramural (most common, respond best to UAE), and submucosal/intracavitary (may pass after UAE).
- Hormonal therapy with intramuscular leuprolide induces menopause via a low-estrogen state by turning off the pituitary secretion of gonadotropins (gonadotropin releasing hormone agonist). It may be used to shrink fibroids before myomectomy or hysterectomy. It has many side effects, which reverse 3 months after withdrawal.
- Myomectomy does not address the entire fibroid burden but is still an option to maintain fertility in younger patients. The failure rate is as high as 40% at 2 years after surgery.
- Hysterectomy requires a 4- to 6-week recovery period, has a high morbidity rate (5–20%), and is associated with loss of fertility.
- Embolization causes the hyaline degeneration of the fibroids while sparing the smaller vessels that supply the normal uterine wall. Average shrinkage is 60%. The clinical success rate for menorrhagia is 81 to 94%, and for bulk symptoms 92 to 96%. Recovery is shorter and the failure rate lower than after surgery.

■ Other Imaging Findings

- Ultrasound: fibroids can be hypoechoic or mixed in a heterogeneous uterus.
- Magnetic resonance imaging (MRI): Fibroids are of low signal intensity on T1- and T2-weighted images and enhance. MRI may better demonstrate pedunculated subserosal fibroids.
- Computed tomography is used for evaluating for postprocedure complications, not for screening. Fibroids often retain air and contrast in the first week after UAE.

✔ Pearls & ✗ Pitfalls

- ✔ Pre-procedure: interventional radiology consultation, evaluation by gynecologist, pelvic ultrasound or MRI.
- ✔ Procedure: Foley catheter, antibiotics, pelvic angiography, embolization of each uterine artery with particles (polyvinyl alcohol or tris-acryl gel spheres). Use Gelfoam (temporary agent) for postpartum hemorrhage. Use microcatheters and nitroglycerin for vasospasm.
- ✔ Post-procedure: patient-controlled analgesia and antiemetics overnight, and oral pain medications at discharge.
- ✗ Abdominal pain lasts 1 to 3 days and tapers by day 5.
- ✗ Sloughing of submucosal fibroids and minor bleeding may occur in the weeks after embolization.
- ✗ Postembolization syndrome (fever, leukocytosis, nausea, and vomiting) may be indistinguishable from infection, and patients may require hospitalization for treatment with intravenous antibiotics.
- ✗ Patients may still require hysterectomy because of complications or clinical failure of embolization (< 2%).
- ✗ Complications include infection, infertility or early menopause, and nontarget embolization.
- ✗ The mortality rate is < 1 per 5000.

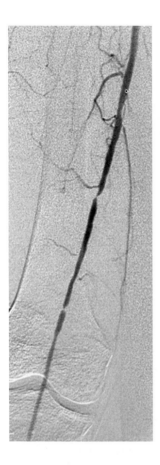

Clinical Presentation

A 70-year-old woman with a 20-year history of smoking presents with intermittent claudication. Her ankle–brachial index is 0.4.

■ Imaging Findings

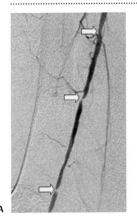 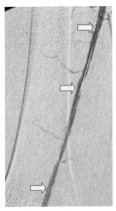

A   B

(A) Conventional angiogram showing three tandem superficial femoral artery stenoses (*arrows*). **(B)** Repeat angiogram showing reduction of stenoses after balloon angioplasty (*arrows*).

■ Differential Diagnosis

- **Superficial femoral artery stenosis:** Indicated by multiple foci of luminal narrowing; the angiographic pattern is typical for atherosclerotic disease.

■ Essential Facts

- A nonimaging diagnosis is based on the history (claudication, pain at rest), physical examination findings (tissue loss, gangrene), and ankle–brachial index (ratio of ankle systolic pressure to brachial systolic pressure: 1.0, normal; 0.3–0.5, severe claudication; < 0.3, pain at rest).
- Stages are claudication, pain at rest, tissue loss, and gangrene according to the Rutherford classification.
- Medical treatment for patients with intermittent claudication who do not require revascularization includes exercise and behavior modification (control of smoking, diabetes, and hyperlipidemia).
- Surgical treatment involves bypass grafts (femoral-to-popliteal, femoral-to-distal [below the knee], or axillary-to-popliteal in severe cases).
- Endovascular treatment includes percutaneous transluminal angioplasty (PTA), stent placement, directional atherectomy, cryoplasty, cutting balloons, covered stents, and drug-eluting stents. The 5-year patency rates range from 16 to 70%, with poorer outcomes for patients with tandem, complex, long, or occlusive lesions and for patients with single-vessel runoff.
- PTA is the treatment of choice for short (< 10 cm), simple femoropopliteal stenosis.
- Stents are usually reserved for long and complex lesions, occlusions, flow-limiting dissection, suboptimal PTA (30% stenosis, 10% systolic gradient), rupture, or pseudoaneurysm (use covered stent).

■ Other Imaging Findings

- Doppler ultrasound shows progression of disease from triphasic (normal) to biphasic (moderate) to monophasic (severe) with gradual loss of amplitude.
- Multidetector computed tomographic angiography (CTA) replaces diagnostic angiography for screening in most cases (100 mL of contrast, 4–5 mL/s, acquired 0.9 mm thick, spaced 0.5 mm; reconstruct maximum-intensity projections and three-dimensional shaded-surface images).

✔ Pearls & ✘ Pitfalls

- ✔ Drugs: 5000 U of heparin before lesion is crossed, 100 µg of nitroglycerin for vasospasm, aspirin and/or clopidogrel for 6 months after the procedure (antiplatelet therapy).
- ✔ Approach: contralateral approach is most common (crossover sheath), but ipsilateral, antegrade puncture is an alternative.
- ✔ After revascularization, repeat angiograms through sheath, maintaining wire access in case of rupture or dissection.
- ✔ Self-expanding nitinol stents remain patent longer (5-year patency rate of 50–60%).
- ✘ Complications include bleeding and pseudoaneurysm at the puncture or treatment site.
- ✘ Distal embolization is more common with occlusions and can sometimes be treated with aspiration thrombectomy. Thrombolysis may be unsuccessful because of the cholesterol content of emboli.
- ✘ Avoid placing balloon-expandable stents in the leg because they deform with mild trauma.

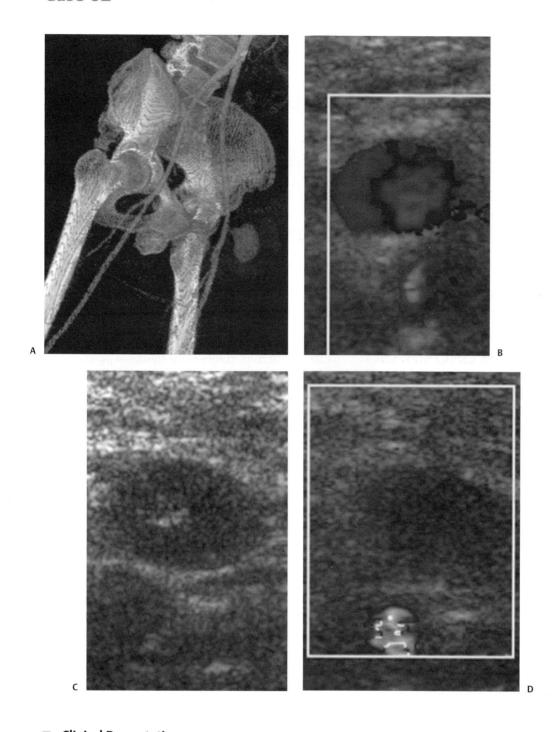

Clinical Presentation

A 51-year-old man presents with swelling in the left groin 2 days after catheterization of the left common femoral artery.

▪ Imaging Findings

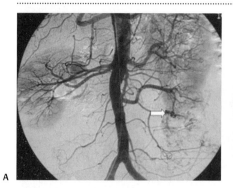 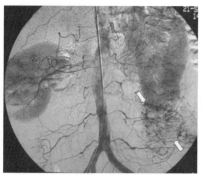

(A) Aortogram shows tortuous arterial branches (*arrow*) below the lower pole of the left kidney. **(B)** Delayed view shows tumor vascularity at this location (*arrows*). No arteriovenous (a-v) shunting is seen.

▪ Differential Diagnosis

- **Angiomyolipoma (AML):** Indicated by hypervascularity with tortuous, dilated arteries and the absence of a-v shunting.
- *Renal cell carcinoma (RCC):* Often uniformly hypervascular with a-v shunting.
- *Metastasis:* May be indistinguishable from RCC and AML by conventional angiogram. CT should be obtained to demonstrate fat components distinguishing AML from malignancy.

▪ Essential Facts

- AMLs are benign hamartomas containing fat, smooth muscle, and vascular tissue. They account for < 3% of renal masses.
- Seventy percent of AMLs are sporadic (typically unilateral and solitary).
- Eighty percent of patients with tuberous sclerosis have AMLs (typically bilateral).
- Embolization is performed for life-threatening bleeding, pain, or symptoms of mass effect. AMLs > 4 cm are embolized because 90% are symptomatic and 50% bleed. The recurrence rate is 30%, and recurrence is often years after embolization.
- Nephron-sparing surgery may replace embolization in cases of severe, life-threatening bleeding.
- The differential diagnosis for a hypervascular renal mass also includes oncocytoma and adenoma. Oncocytoma may have a "spoked wheel" appearance of arterial branching.

▪ Other Imaging Findings

- A contrast-enhanced computed tomographic (CT) scan showing macroscopic fat in a renal mass is virtually diagnostic of AML. CT also measures the size of AMLs and reveals hemorrhage.
- Conventional renal angiography is typically performed with intent to embolize. Active extravasation is rare, but embolization of feeders is still performed. Findings include tumor vascularity, ectatic vessels, and bizarre aneurysms.
- In benign tumors of the kidney, a-v shunting is typically absent.

✔ Pearls & ✘ Pitfalls

- ✔ Superselective catheterization of arterial feeders is performed (with a microcatheter if necessary).
- ✔ Alcohol or particles (polyvinyl alcohol or gel spheres) are the preferred agents. Coils are ineffective because of collateral flow.
- ✔ If you inject alcohol, maintain arterial stasis with a balloon occlusion catheter to avoid nontarget embolization.
- ✘ Complications include nontarget embolization, reduction of renal function (although the risk may be worse with surgical resection), and arterial injury.

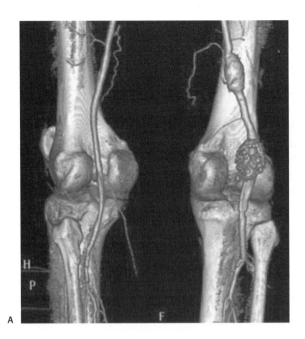

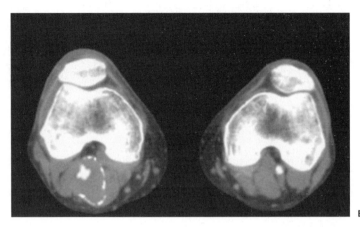

A

B

■ Clinical Presentation

A 48-year-old man presents to the emergency department with a cold right foot.

■ Imaging Findings

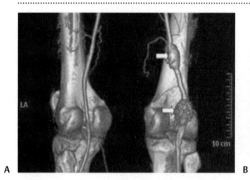
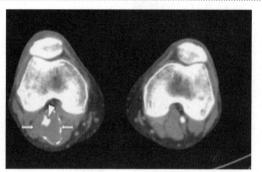

(A) Computed tomographic angiogram (CTA) shows large aneurysms in the right superficial femoral and popliteal arteries (*arrows*). **(B)** Axial images show extensive intraluminal thrombus narrowing the lumen (*arrowhead*); conventional angiography underestimates the aneurysmal size (*arrows*).

■ Differential Diagnosis

- **Popliteal artery aneurysm (PAA):** Indicated by fusiform dilatation > 1.2 cm and at least 1.5 times the luminal diameter of the proximal arterial segment.
- *Vascular ectasia:* Would be indicated by a dilated PA without frank PAA.

■ Essential Facts

- PAA is the most common type of peripheral artery aneurysm; it is more common in male patients, bilateral in 50% of cases, and often associated with aortoiliac aneurysms. These lesions rarely rupture.
- Symptomatic patients present with a cold foot or leg resulting from acute thrombosis or distal embolization; asymptomatic patients present with a pulsatile popliteal mass on physical examination.
- For symptomatic patients, treatment is strongly encouraged because two thirds will experience acute lower extremity ischemia over a 5-year period.
- For asymptomatic patients, treatment of PAAs > 2 cm in diameter is recommended; intraluminal thrombus and poor distal runoff have been identified as risk factors for future complications.
- Thrombolysis is usually performed before bypass or endovascular repair for patients presenting with acute ischemia in a viable limb. Catheter-directed infusion of a recombinant tissue–type plasminogen activator (rt-PA) treats acute popliteal thrombosis and distal embolization.
- Surgical repair consists of ligation and bypass.
- Endovascular stent-graft placement is associated with less blood loss and with a shorter procedure time and hospital stay than is surgical repair. The advantages of stent-grafts must be weighed against their slightly lower patency rates versus those of surgical repair.

■ Other Imaging Findings

- Doppler ultrasonography is a fast screening tool that can distinguish PAAs from other masses in the popliteal fossa. Because up to one third of patients with PAAs repaired by surgical or endovascular techniques will require a secondary intervention, surveillance with Doppler improves limb salvage and secondary patency.
- Multidetector CT with CTA provides information for treatment planning, such as the location of associated peripheral artery disease, the position of branches to avoid type 2 endoleaks, and the size of the PAA for stent-graft selection. Evaluate source images when determining vessel patency; three-dimensional images can underestimate diameter as a consequence of mural thrombus.
- Magnetic resonance angiography is an alternative to CTA.
- Conventional angiography is used to guide endovascular treatment but has largely been replaced by Doppler ultrasonography and CTA for diagnosis and treatment planning.

✔ Pearls & ✘ Pitfalls

- ✔ The largest prospective studies of endovascular repair of PAAs involve the use of nitinol stents covered with polytetrafluoroethylene (PTFE).
- ✔ Antiplatelet therapy (aspirin and/or clopiderol) is recommended following stent placement.
- ✔ Patency rates for stent-grafts are similar or slightly inferior to those associated with open surgical repair (primary, 80–87% at 1 year and 77% at 2 years; secondary, 90–100% at 1 year and 87% at 2 years).
- ✔ Patency rates for surgical bypass (primary patency) are as high as 100% at 1 year, > 90% for asymptomatic patients at 5 years, and > 75% for symptomatic patients at 5 years.
- ✘ The disadvantage of endovascular repair is limited flexibility of stent-grafts placed in a location subject to constant flexion and extension.
- ✘ Major and minor complications have been reported in up to 37% of stent-grafts, including migration, endoleak with continued enlargement of the aneurysm, stenosis at the edge of the stent-graft, and stent breakage.

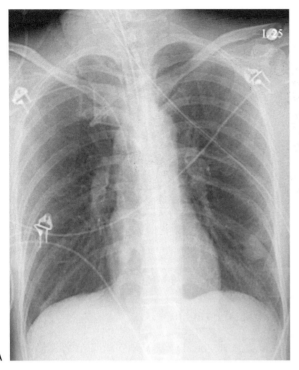

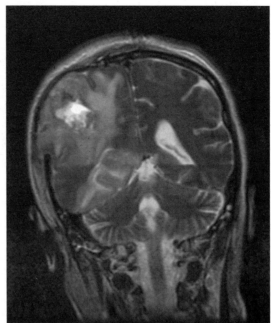

Clinical Presentation

A 37-year-old woman presents with hemiplegia.

■ Imaging Findings

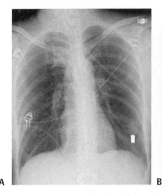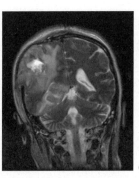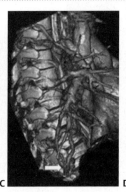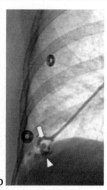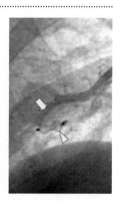

A   B   C   D   E

(A) Chest radiograph shows a well-circumscribed mass in the left lower lobe (*arrow*). **(B)** Magnetic resonance image shows a ring-enhancing lesion in the right hemisphere with mass effect. **(C)** Follow-up computed tomographic angiogram (CTA) shows an arteriovenous (a-v) malformation in the right lower lobe (*arrow*). Other a-v malformations were present bilat-
erally. **(D)** Selected pulmonary arteriogram shows artery (*arrow*) and vein (*arrowhead*) of the a-v malformation. **(E)** Repeat angiogram shows stasis in artery (*arrow*) supplying angiogram after deployment of an occluding device (*arrowhead*).

■ Differential Diagnosis

- *Pulmonary arteriovenous malformation:* Suggested by vessels associated with a smoothly marginated nodule coupled with a brain lesion suspected to be an abscess resulting from a paradoxical embolus.
- *Primary lung cancer or metastatic disease:* May present as a smoothly marginated nodule with a ring-enhancing brain metastasis.

■ Essential Facts

- The transmission of hereditary hemorrhagic telangectasia (HHT), also known as *Osler-Weber-Rendu disease,* is autosomal-dominant. The incidence is 2 per 100,000. HHT typically occurs in young patients.
- Twenty percent of patients with HHT have simple pulmonary a-v malformations—usually a single artery to single draining vein, whereas 80% of patients with pulmonary a-v malformations have HHT.
- Symptoms may include respiratory dysfunction, hemoptysis, high-output cardiac failure, or paradoxical thromboembolus from pulmonary arteries through the AVM to pulmonary veins, and then to systemic arteries causing symptoms of stroke or brain abscess. More than 75% of primarily discovered a-v malformations may be asymptomatic.
- Paradoxical embolus may present with stroke, brain abscess, myocardial infarction, mesenteric infarction, or peripheral artery thromboembolus.
- The differential diagnosis includes hepatopulmonary syndrome in patients with cirrhosis, who may present with a-v malformations of a lower lobe.
- Pulmonary angiography with embolization of the arterial supply is the definitive treatment in almost all cases. Agents include coils, detachable balloons, and other large vessel occlusion devices. Never use temporary agents (Gelfoam recanalizes and results in recurrence) or particles (these paradoxically embolize to the systemic arteries).

■ Other Imaging Findings

- Plain radiographs typically show well-circumscribed, non-calcified nodules, more commonly in the lower lobes.
- Multidetector CTA identifies the pulmonary arterial supply and pulmonary venous drainage to verify the diagnosis and plan treatment. Look for the size and number of arteries supplying the a-v malformation and for additional a-v malformations.
- Conventional angiography is undertaken with the intent to perform transarterial embolization.

✔ Pearls & ✘ Pitfalls

- ✔ Those a-v malformations with arterial supply > 3 mm in diameter are treated, but many radiologists embolize all visible a-v malformations because of the risk for interval enlargement (see below).
- ✔ All arterial feeders must be embolized to complete hemostasis to prevent recurrence.
- ✔ The technical success rate is > 96%.
- ✔ Patients who have HHT are often treated with prophylactic antibiotics because of the risk for brain abscess.
- ✘ Complications of embolization of pulmonary a-v malformations include paradoxical coil embolus (< 1%) and air embolus to the coronary arteries (< 5%).
- ✘ Recurrence after embolization (3%) is typically caused by recanalization of the embolized artery or accessory feeding arteries (pulmonary or bronchial). Recurrent a-v malformations are more likely to be symptomatic.
- ✘ Interval enlargement of small, untreated a-v malformations over 3 to 7 years has been documented by serial CT studies in patients with HHT, so many advocate regular CT examinations and a low threshold for embolizing enlarging a-v malformations.

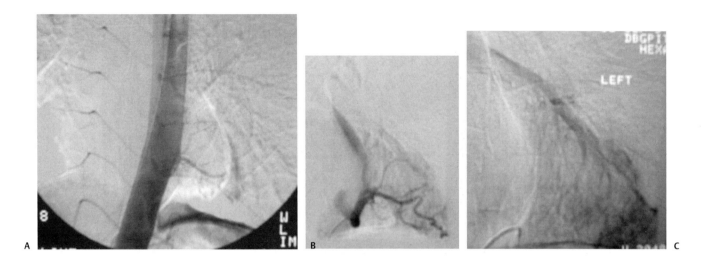

■ Clinical Presentation

A 35-year-old man presents with fever, chronic shortness of breath, and occasional hemoptysis.

■ Imaging Findings

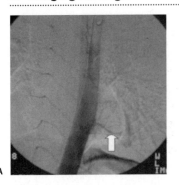 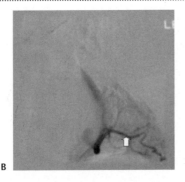 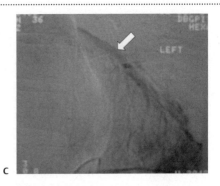

(A) Thoracic angiogram shows a small vessel (*arrow*) off the aorta, just above the left hemidiaphragm. **(B)** Selected angiogram of this vessel shows branches (*arrow*) supplying a region of the left lower lobe. **(C)** Venous phase shows pulmonary venous (*arrow*) drainage.

■ Differential Diagnosis

- **Intralobar pulmonary sequestration:** Indicated by a left lower lobe structure with systemic artery supply and pulmonary venous drainage.

■ Essential Facts

- Sequestration likely arises as an abnormality of foregut development during the first 2 months of embryogenesis that results in a separate lung bud supplied by anomalous systemic arteries and lacking normal bronchial communication.
- Intralobar sequestrations (ILS) lack a separate pleural membrane and are more common than extralobar sequestrations (ELS). ILS occur on the left side in 60% of cases.
- Venous drainage is via the pulmonary veins in 95% of cases.
- ILS show no sexual predominance and present later in life than do ELS because of the near-absence of associated congenital anomalies.
- Symptoms are related to chronic pulmonary infections, high-output cardiac failure, and bleeding.
- ELS have a separate pleural membrane, most commonly occur on the left side between the lung and diaphragm, and may occur in the chest, diaphragm, or abdomen.
- Venous drainage is via the systemic veins in 75% (25% with some pulmonary venous drainage).
- ELS are more common in male patients and usually present in the first 6 months of life as a consequence of associated anomalies.
- Symptoms may be respiratory, gastrointestinal, and/or cardiac in association with hypoplastic lung, congenital lobar emphysema, congenital cystic adenomatoid malformation, bronchogenic cyst, diaphragmatic hernia (most common association), enteric duplication cysts, total anomalous pulmonary venous return, truncus arteriosus, dextrocardia, and pericardial defects.

■ Other Imaging Findings

- Plain radiographs may show a subtle opacity, often in the left lower lobe and often partially obscured by the cardiac silhouette. For ELS, look for associated anomalies and azygos enlargement due to anomalous systemic venous drainage.
- Multidetector computed tomographic angiography or magnetic resonance imaging/angiography may show a homogeneous or inhomogeneous mass, a solid component mimicking neoplasm, cysts with air and fluid, and emphysema in the adjacent lung. For ELS, look for associated anomalies and azygos enlargement.
- Conventional angiography shows systemic arterial supply to a dense, focal blush. Venous drainage usually distinguishes ELS from ILS.

✔ Pearls & ✗ Pitfalls

- ✔ The treatment of sequestrations is usually surgical resection, although embolization has been described.
- ✔ Asymptomatic, untreated sequestrations can lead to respiratory infections, gastroesophageal reflux, and asthma, emphasizing the need for follow-up.
- ✔ Some physicians recommend surgery only when complications are detected. Others recommend aggressive early intervention.
- ✗ The anomalous vascularity of sequestrations may be confused with arteriovenous (a-v) malformations or neoplasms. Pulmonary a-v malformations are usually of the simple type—single pulmonary artery to pulmonary vein.
- ✗ Complications of embolization have included pain and pleural effusion.

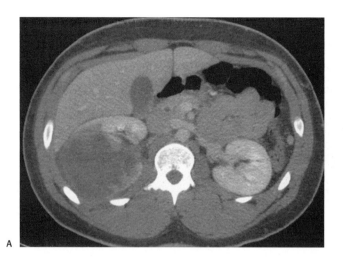

A

■ Clinical Presentation

A 19-year-old man presents to the emergency department with sepsis. A second study is obtained 3 weeks after catheter placement.

Further Work-up

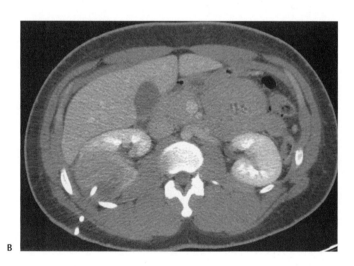

B

■ Imaging Findings

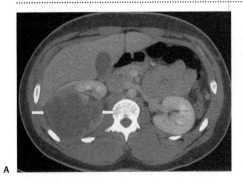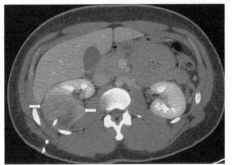

A   B

(A) A contrast-enhanced computed tomographic (CT) scan shows a low-density collection in the right kidney (*arrows*). **(B)** Three weeks after drain placement, there is a persistent, large, low-density area despite low output in an afebrile patient (*arrows*).

■ Differential Diagnosis

- ***Drain placed in a clear cell sarcoma:*** The lack of complete resolution on imaging studies should prompt consideration of causes of refractory fluid collections.

■ Essential Facts

- Refractory collections that remain despite placement of a drainage catheter include tumors, viscous collections, organizing hematomas, and collections that have formed a fistula or are connected to fluid-producing structures.
- "Do not drain" collections typically include tumors, acute hematomas, and those associated with acute bowel rupture and peritonitis. Surgical treatment is usually required.
- Infected tumors may require drain placement in patients with sepsis when there is no surgical option.
- Viscous collections and organizing hematomas may require drain upsizing and/or fibrinolysis with 4 to 6 mg of a recombinant tissue–type plasminogen activator in 20 to 50 mL of saline incubated in the collection for 4 to 6 hours and then withdrawn.
- Fistulas may develop from an abscess to bowel, bile duct, pancreatic duct, or urinary tract.
- Fistulas from abscess to bowel may close spontaneously with long-term drainage of the abscess and bowel rest. Fibrin glue has been used with variable success.
- Fistulas from abscess to urinary tract may require urinary diversion with nephrostomy tube placement to facilitate healing.
- Fistulas from hepatic abscess to bile ducts are often caused by biliary ischemia and may be refractory to external drainage. Biliary drain placement may be necessary for bile diversion to facilitate healing.

■ Other Imaging Findings

- Contrast-enhanced CT features suggesting tumor over abscess include enhancing nodular components and additional enhancing lesions.
- Abscessogram (contrast injection under fluoroscopy) is indicated if continued, nontapering output from a catheter suggests a fistula.

✔ Pearls & ✘ Pitfalls

- ✔ In aseptic patients, consider core biopsy or aspiration for cytology to rule out tumor before catheter drainage.
- ✔ Repeat imaging may be required if clinical improvement does not occur despite drain placement, even when output has tapered. A refractory loculated or viscous component should be suspected.
- ✔ Low-output fistulas (colonic) heal in weeks, but high-output fistulas (small bowel, 200 mL/d) heal in months, and patients often require the combination of bowel rest and parenteral nutrition.
- ✘ Both tumors and abscesses can have an enhancing rim, making them indistinguishable by contrast-enhanced studies.
- ✘ Seeding of the percutaneous access tract has been described for drains placed in tumors.
- ✘ Once tumors are drained, drain removal may not be possible because of a lack of normal tissue around the catheter insertion site to facilitate healing.

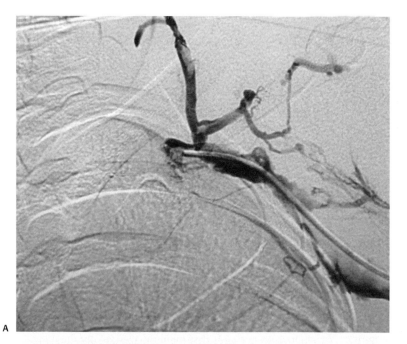

A

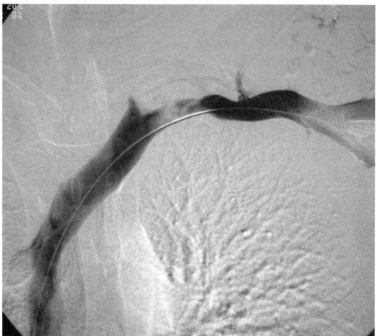

B

■ Clinical Presentation

A 31-year-old man presents with marked pain and swelling of the left arm.

■ Imaging Findings

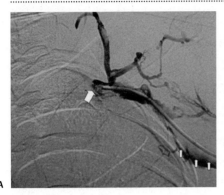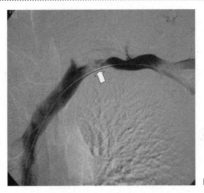

A   B

(A) Left upper extremity venography shows complete occlusion (*large arrow*) of the subclavian vein at the thoracic outlet and intraluminal thrombus (*small arrows*) in the axillary and subclavian veins. **(B)** Venography after thrombolysis shows stenosis at the thoracic inlet (*arrow*).

■ Differential Diagnosis

- ***Paget von Schroetter syndrome (PSS):*** Indicated by complete subclavian vein occlusion at the thoracic outlet with associated intraluminal thrombus.

■ Essential Facts

- PSS is also known as *effort thrombosis* of the axillary or subclavian veins at the thoracic inlet. Narrowing without thrombosis is venous *thoracic outlet syndrome*. The cause is compression at the thoracic outlet by structures such as the first rib, the anterior scalene muscle, the costoclavicular ligament, cervical ribs, and exostoses.
- Patients are usually in their mid-30s with a slight male predominance.
- Symptoms include arm swelling, exercise fatigue, and pain.
- Treatment typically involves both endovascular and surgical procedures.
- The endovascular treatment of PSS requires catheter-directed thrombolysis: a low dose of recombinant tissue–type plasminogen activator (e.g., 0.5 mg/h) over 1 to 2 days with a subtherapeutic infusion of heparin through a separate sheath or intravenous line (< 500 U/h).
- Angioplasty or stent placement is performed after surgical decompression in cases with fixed venous defects, such as tight stenoses, webs, or senechiae.
- Surgical treatment is performed after successful thrombolysis. The most common procedure is resection of the first rib via the transaxillary approach and release of the anterior scalene muscle. In severe cases, resection of the costoclavicular ligament or a portion of the clavicle is required. Debilitating cases may require axillojugular bypass or anastomosis.

■ Other Imaging Findings

- Duplex scanning serves as a noninvasive, first-line test and a follow-up test after treatment. Images are obtained in neutral and hyperabducted (stressed) arm positions. Positive results can also be seen in asymptomatic patients and must be correlated with the clinical symptoms.
- Radiography may identify a bony cause of venous obstruction, such as a cervical rib or exostosis.
- Venography provides further evaluation of suggestive findings. In patients with PSS, the extent of central venous thrombosis can be identified and catheter-directed thrombolysis initiated. For thoracic inlet syndrome, complete obstruction of the subclavian vein is identified by venography during hyperabduction.

✔ Pearls & ✘ Pitfalls

- ✔ Treatment of PSS within 1 month after the onset of symptoms usually results in complete recovery. Delayed or no treatment can result in chronic disability.
- ✔ Clinical success rates of endovascular treatment are good to excellent in 89% of cases, fair in 11%.
- ✘ Complications of endovascular treatments include acute recurrence of axillary vein thrombosis (< 24 hours) requiring repeat intervention, hematomas around the sheath, and minor bleeding. No deaths, pulmonary embolus, cerebral hemorrhage, or other major bleeding complications have been reported.
- ✘ Technical failure (0–15%) increases with the extent and chronicity of thrombosis.

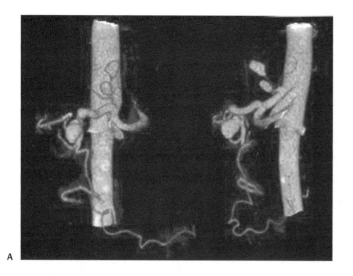

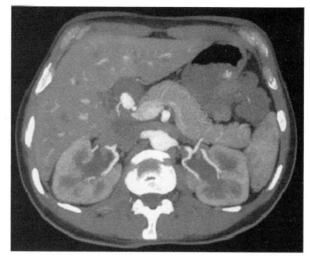

A

B

Clinical Presentation

An elderly man presents with abdominal pain.

Further Work-up

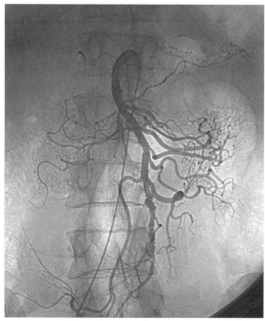

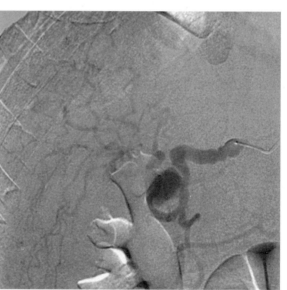

C

D

■ **Imaging Findings**

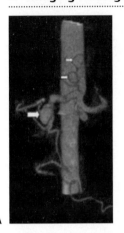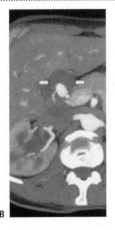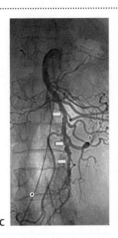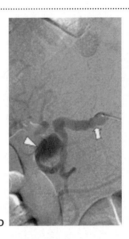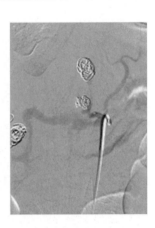

A B C D E

(A) Three-dimensional volume-rendered computed tomographic angiogram (CTA) shows saccular aneurysms of the hepatic (*large arrow*) and left gastric (*small arrows*) arteries. **(B)** Contrast-enhanced CT scan shows a thrombosed component of the hepatic artery aneurysm (*arrows*). **(C)** Selected superior mesenteric artery angiogram shows diffuse beading and fo-cal segments of dilatation (*arrows*). **(D)** Selected hepatic angiogram shows beading of the common hepatic artery (*arrow*) and aneurysm of the proper hepatic artery (*arrowhead*). **(E)** Selected celiac angiogram shows successful coil embolization of the left gastric and hepatic aneurysms.

■ **Differential Diagnosis**

- ***Segmental arterial mediolysis (SAM):*** Indicated by predominantly celiac branch involvement.
- *Fibromuscular dysplasia:* Suggested by beading of the superior mesenteric artery.
- *Mycotic pseudoaneurysms:* Typically sacular.
- *Vasculitis:* Such as giant cell or Takayasu's arteritis may present with aneurysms.

■ **Essential Facts**

- SAM is a rare disorder that usually affects the elderly and is fatal in > 50% of patients in the acute phase.
- Locations: SAM most commonly involves the celiac arterial distribution; less commonly affected are the superior and inferior mesenteric arteries and the renal arteries.
- Symptoms include the following: abdominal pain from dissection or thrombosis with bowel ischemia; hypotension, distension, or anemia from gastrointestinal or peritoneal hemorrhage secondary to aneurysm rupture.
- The acute phase is characterized by the deposition of fibrin and collagen in the media without an inflammatory infiltrate.
- The late phase is characterized by reparative remodeling of the vessel wall.
- Treatment options include the following: coil embolization of aneurysms to prevent rupture; surgical bypass or thrombectomy (depending on the cause of occlusion).

■ **Other Imaging Findings**

- Acute phase angiography (CTA, magnetic resonance angiography, or conventional) shows segments of arterial dilatation, narrowing, and beading. Occlusion may result from thrombosis, dissection, or stricture. Aneurysms may rupture or erode adjacent structures, such as bile ducts, bowel, and peritoneum.
- Late phase angiography (delayed 6 months) shows resolution of beading and dilatation, often leaving a smooth arterial wall.

✔ **Pearls & ✗ Pitfalls**

- ✔ Unlike FMD, SAM shows a predilection for the celiac distribution, has a high rate of mortality from aneurysmal rupture and bowel ischemia, undergoes spontaneous repair and remodeling, and is typically not treated with angioplasty.
- ✔ Unlike vasculitis, SAM is not associated with inflammatory infiltration and does not respond to steroids and immunosuppressants.
- ✔ Unlike mycotic aneurysms, the aneurysms of SAM are not typically associated with arterial branch points.
- ✗ Complications of coil embolization include arterial dissection, rupture, and thrombosis resulting from nontarget embolization or clot propagation.
- ✗ Saccular aneurysms are usually amenable to embolization, but fusiform aneurysms may require ligation and bypass. Stent-grafts may play an increasing role.

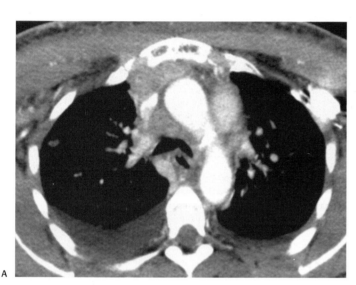

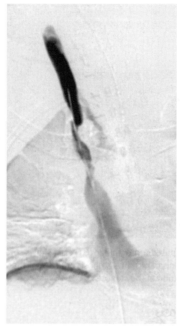

A

B

Clinical Presentation

A 49-year-old woman with a history of metastatic breast cancer presents with facial swelling and shortness of breath.

■ **Imaging Findings**

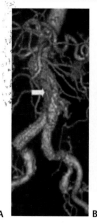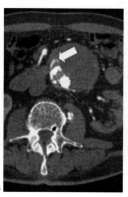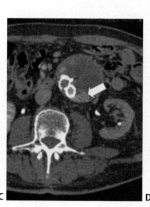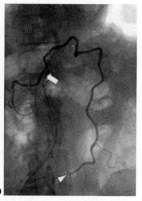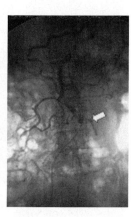

A   B   C   D   E

(A) Three-dimensional volume-rendered computed tomographic angiogram (CTA) shows stent-graft in place to treat infrarenal aortic aneurysm. The density anterior to the graft (*arrow*) represents leakage of contrast into excluded aneurysm. **(B,C)** Arterial and delayed phase axial CT images show contrast within the aneurysm sac (*arrows*). **(D)** After selection of the super-ior mesenteric artery (SMA: *arrow*), the middle colic artery was subselected, and angiography shows filling of the inferior mesenteric artery (IMA: *arrowhead*), which supplies the aneurysm. **(E)** From the SMA approach, the IMA origin is embolized through a microcatheter with coils (*arrow*).

■ **Differential Diagnosis**

• ***Type 2 endoleak:*** This is the only diagnosis, indicated by the IMA supply to the aneurysm sac.

■ **Essential Facts**

• Definition: In patients with stent-grafts, an endoleak occurs when blood flow persists outside the endograft but within the aneurysm sac or adjacent, communicating arterial branch. This leads to continued arterial pressure in the sac, continued expansion, and increased risk for rupture.
• Type 2 endoleak indicates filling of the sac by inflow and outflow vessels originating from the aneurysm, such as the inferior mesenteric and lumbar arteries.
• CTA is the modality of choice for the detection of endoleaks and for serial follow-up of the aneurysm size, and it should be performed in three phases: unenhanced, arterially weighted, and delayed. Unenhanced scans are necessary because calcification can be mistaken for endoleak, and delayed scans are needed to detect some type 2 leaks that slowly perfuse the sac.
• Embolization is the first-line treatment for type 2 endoleaks; it is performed via catheter subselection or translumbar puncture of the aneurysm. Agents include coils to occlude branch vessels and glue or thrombin to induce thrombosis of the sac.

■ **Other Imaging Findings**

• Doppler ultrasound is a rapid, noninvasive, inexpensive means to assess aneurysm size. Limitations include decreased sensitivity and operator variability for serial surveillance studies.
• Conventional angiography is usually performed with the intent to embolize the feeding artery.

✔ **Pearls & ✘ Pitfalls**

✔ Catheterization of the SMA allows superselection of the IMA with a microcatheter and embolization with microcoils.
✔ Translumbar puncture and injection of the aneurysm sac can be performed to demonstrate and embolize difficult feeding vessels such as lumbar arteries.
✔ Type 2 endoleaks may resolve spontaneously and not lead to sac expansion. Serial CT may prove stability and obviate the need for treatment.
✔ The translumbar approach is currently favored as the best technique for type 2 endoleak embolization because the success rate is higher than with the transfemoral subselection of feeding arteries.
✘ Type 2 endoleaks must be distinguished from other types by imaging studies (see Case 80 for classification).
✘ Complications of embolization of type 2 endoleaks include nontarget embolization, mesenteric thrombosis, and sac hemorrhage.

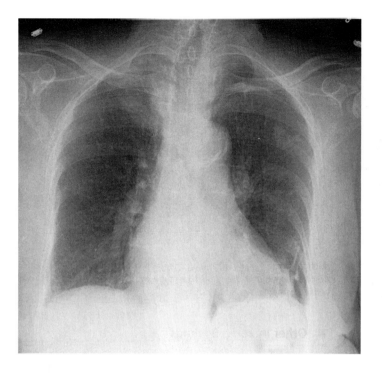

■ Clinical Presentation

An 88-year-old woman reports chest pain after chest biopsy.

■ Imaging Findings

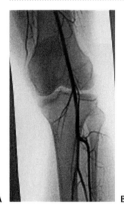
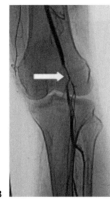

(A) Conventional angiogram in neutral dorsiflexion is normal. **(B)** Conventional angiogram in stressed plantar flexion shows occlusion of the popliteal artery above the knee (*arrow*) with reconstitution by small collateral arteries.

■ Differential Diagnosis

- ***Popliteal artery entrapment syndrome (PAES):*** Indicated by focal popliteal occlusion seen only during plantar flexion view.
- *Cystic adventitial disease:* Results in occlusion and loss of the distal pulses during knee flexion rather than plantar flexion and may progress to fixed arterial occlusion.
- *Thrombosed popliteal artery aneurysm:* May cause popliteal occlusion and is unlikely to be transient and positional, as in this case.
- *Thromboembolism and vasospasm:* These are always considerations for sudden arterial occlusion during conventional angiography. Thrombosis would occlude the more distal arteries, and vasospasm is more common in the smaller, infrapopliteal arteries with catheter manipulation.

■ Essential Facts

- PAES is extrinsic compression of the popliteal artery (PA) due to its abnormal position in relationship to the surrounding structures.
- Its incidence is unknown, but it is very uncommon. The condition is bilateral in 25% of patients, who are typically adults between the ages of 20 and 40 years; 75 to 85% are male.
- Risk factors include occupational or athletic activities that develop the leg muscles and enhance the compressive effect.
- The presentation is intermittent calf claudication in the majority of cases; acute ischemia from thromboembolus is less common.
- Types:
  1. Aberrant course of the PA medial to and deep to the medial head of the gastrocnemius muscle.
  2. Normal course of the PA; compression is by the medial head of gastrocnemius, which arises on the intercondylar area rather than the medial epicondyle.
  3. An aberrant extra musculotendinous slip of the medial head of the gastrocnemius arising from the intercondylar area compresses the PA.

  4. The PA passes deep to the popliteus muscle and medial head of the gastrocnemius (most common).
  5. Entrapment includes the popliteal vein.
- The natural progression is toward associated abnormalities, including premature atherosclerosis, aneurysm, stenosis, occlusion, and thromboembolism.
- The treatment is surgical decompression with or without revascularization to correct arterial sequelae.

■ Other Imaging Findings

- Imaging studies and a physical examination should be performed in the unstressed (dorsiflexion) and stressed (plantar flexion) positions.
- Duplex scanning showing loss of the normal triphasic waveform is often used as a screening tool, but patients with well-developed calf muscles and no PAES may exhibit PA compression on dorsiflexion.
- Conventional arteriography is the best study of the associated intrinsic arterial pathology and distal thromboembolus. Medial deviation of the popliteal artery is diagnostic of PAES, but not always demonstrated. It does not identify myofascial structures causing compression.
- Magnetic resonance angiography or computed tomographic angiography provides angiographic images of the popliteal artery and distal runoff vessels in addition to a three-dimensional evaluation of myofascial structures causing compression.

✔ Pearls & ✗ Pitfalls

- ✔ PAES should be strongly considered in all symptomatic young male athletes unlikely to have an alternative cause of lower extremity ischemia.
- ✗ PAES refers to symptomatic patients with associated imaging findings. Imaging studies may be positive during plantar flexion in patients with well-developed calf muscles and no PAES.

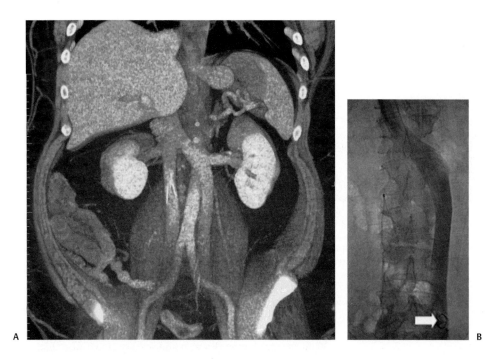

A   B

■ Clinical Presentation

A patient presents with gastrointestinal bleeding, deep venous thrombosis (DVT), and recurrent pulmonary embolism (PE) despite caval filtration.

■ Imaging Findings

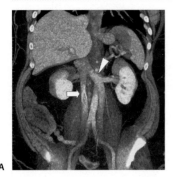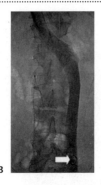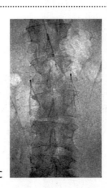

A   B   C

(A) Selected image is a coronal volume slab from an infused computed tomographic (CT) scan shows a filter in a right-sided inferior vena cava (IVC: *arrow*). The IVC is duplicated, with the left component draining into the left renal vein (*arrowhead*). **(B)** Conventional venogram with pigtail (*arrow*) in left component and filter in right component. **(C)** Fluoroscopic image with bilateral filters in place.

■ Differential Diagnosis

- ***Duplicated inferior vena cava***

■ Essential Facts

- Definition: failure of regression of the left supracardinal vein results in two large veins draining the lower extremities—the anomalous left typically draining into the left renal vein or the right IVC at the level of the renal veins.
- The incidence of duplication is < 3%. Anomalies of the renal veins and IVC occur in up to 37% of cases.
- Clinical significance includes a possible predisposition to DVT, the need for bilateral filter placement for protection against PE, and potential injury to the variant left IVC during surgical procedures.
- Recurrent PE despite filter placement may also be associated with duplicated renal veins, suprarenal caval thrombosis, upper extremity or central venous thrombosis, and thromboembolism through an existing filter.
- Caval filtration options for duplicated IVC include bilateral infrarenal caval filters or a single suprarenal caval filter. The first option is preferred because filtration above the level of the renal veins theoretically places the kidneys at risk for renal vein thrombosis.

■ Other Imaging Finding

- Vena cavagram may show an abnormally small infrarenal IVC and absent inflow from the left common iliac vein.

✔ Pearls & ✘ Pitfalls

- ✔ Inability to pass a wire into the left iliac vein during filter placement from a jugular approach may signal duplicated IVC.
- ✔ Other IVC and renal vein anomalies include circumaortic left renal vein, retroaortic left renal vein, multiple left or right renal veins, azygos continuation of the IVC, and congenital megacava.
- ✘ Absent inflow from the left common iliac vein may also occur with left-sided pelvic DVT or with May–Thurner syndrome.
- ✘ Failure to diagnose duplicated IVC may result in injury of the anomalous left IVC during operations involving structures such as the spine, aorta, kidney, and ureter.

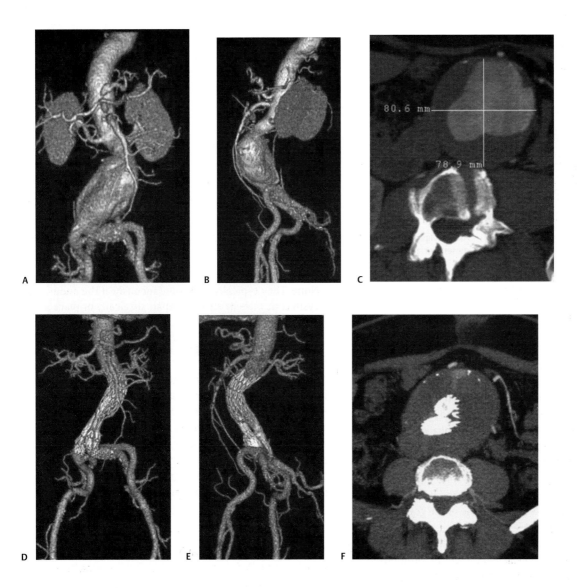

A   B   C

D   E   F

◼ Clinical Presentation

The patient is a 50-year-old who underwent repair of an abdominal aortic aneurysm (AAA).

■ Imaging Findings

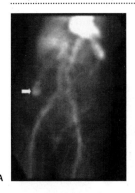 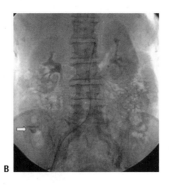 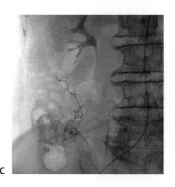 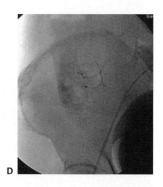

(A) Selected technetium Tc 99m tagged red blood cell (RBC) study shows mobile radioactive tracer in the right hemiabdomen (*arrow*). **(B)** Selected superior mesenteric angiogram shows extravasation in the right lower quadrant (*arrow*). **(C)** Superselected ileocolic branch angiogram with use of a microcatheter. **(D)** Successful embolization of two cecal branches with microcoils.

■ Differential Diagnosis

• *Colonic hemorrhage*

■ Essential Facts

• Common causes are diverticulosis, neoplasia, and angiodysplasia.
• Colonoscopy may be used to diagnose and treat bleeding in acute cases but requires adequate bowel preparation. In many cases, diagnosis and treatment are performed by radiologists.
• A tagged RBC scan is performed to localize and verify active bleeding. Its sensitivity is better than that of angiography because the bleeding may be slow or intermittent, and the scans are performed continuously over hours.
• Angiography and embolization should be carried out within 1 hour if the RBC scan result is positive.
• Superselective embolization (with a microcatheter) is the primary treatment option. The marginal artery or terminal vasa recta may be embolized.
• Embolic agents used include (most commonly) microcoils and Gelfoam. Particles are sometimes used for angiodysplasia.

■ Other Imaging Findings

• Multidetector computed tomographic angiography may replace tagged RBC scan to screen patients for active bleeding.
• All patients with lower gastrointestinal (GI) bleeding should eventually undergo colonoscopy to determine the underlying cause.

✔ Pearls & ✘ Pitfalls

✔ Medical treatment resolves most cases of lower GI bleeding—correction of coagulopathy, fluid resuscitation, transfusion of blood products.
✔ Immediate angiography, with omission of the tagged RBC study, may be necessary in the setting of very brisk bleeding.
✔ Infusion of vasopressin into the mesenteric or celiac artery has largely fallen out of favor because of the ischemic complications and prolonged treatment time. Protocol: 0.2 U/h, increase to 0.4 U/h if unsuccessful, taper over 12 to 24 hours if successful.
✘ Risk for ischemia from superselective colonic embolization is < 5%.
✘ Right-sided colonic bleeding is less responsive to embolization than left-sided colonic bleeding. This is likely caused by a preponderance of angiodysplasia in the right side of the colon, which is less responsive to embolization than predominantly left-sided diverticulosis.
✘ Patients with multifocal disorders such as diverticulosis are at increased risk for recurrent bleeding from other sites.

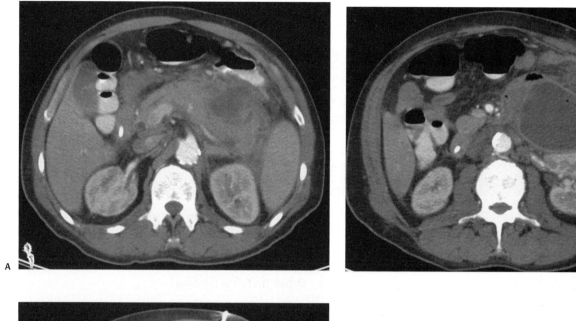

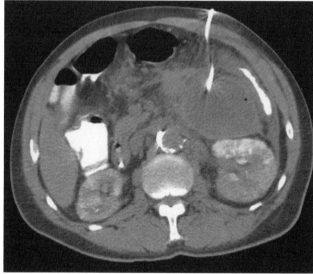

Clinical Presentation

A 46-year-old man presents to the emergency department with fever, nausea, vomiting, and back pain. The image in Figure A was obtained on the day of admission. The images in Figures B and C were obtained 4 weeks later.

■ Imaging Findings

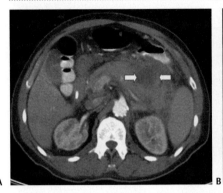
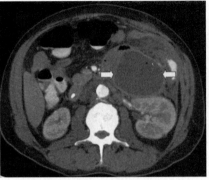
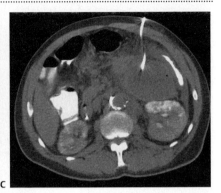

(A) Infused computed tomographic (CT) scan shows fluid collection (*arrows*), fat stranding, and an enlarged pancreas, consistent with acute fluid collection of pancreatitis. **(B)** Image obtained 4 weeks later shows enlarg- ing, painful pseudocyst with a well-defined, enhancing wall (*arrows*). **(C)** A percutaneous drain was placed.

■ Differential Diagnosis

- ***Pancreatic pseudocyst:*** Indicated by development of a walled-off pancreatic collection in 4 weeks.
- *Pancreatic phlegmon:* Presents as a swollen, inflamed pancreas.
- *Pancreatic abscess:* May be indistinguishable from a pseudocyst.

■ Essential Facts

- Pancreatic fluid collections occurring within the first 4 weeks of pancreatitis include acute fluid collections, pancreatic phlegmon and necrosis, and pancreatic abscess.
- Pancreatic fluid collections occurring after 4 weeks include abscesses and pseudocysts.
- Acute pancreatic fluid collections of pancreatitis have no well-defined wall on CT (Fig. A) and typically resolve spontaneously. Needle aspiration may become necessary.
- The term *pancreatic phlegmon and necrosis* describes an enhancing, swollen, inflamed pancreas on CT scan. Catheter drainage usually fails because of a high level of viscosity.
- Pancreatic abscesses have a high mortality rate, so emergent drainage is indicated.
- Pseudocysts have a well-defined wall and contain a mixture of autodigested tissue, pancreatic fluid, and blood.
- Simple pseudocysts commonly resolve without drainage.
- Complicated pseudocysts cause pain, bleeding, or infection, exhibit increased size (> 5 cm) and continuing enlargement, and require drainage.
- Treatment options for pseudocysts include percutaneous drainage, endoscopic cyst-gastrostomy, and surgical cyst-enterostomy.
- Percutaneous routes of drainage are transperitoneal, retroperitoneal, and transgastric.

■ Other Imaging Finding

- Magnetic resonance cholangiopancreatography or endoscopic retrograde cholangiopancreatography is sometimes performed to evaluate duct patency and duct–cyst communication to determine the appropriate treatment of pseudocysts—surgical, endoscopic, or percutaneous drainage.

✔ Pearls & ✘ Pitfalls

- ✔ The duration of percutaneous drainage of pseudocysts is shortest when the cyst does not communicate with the pancreatic duct.
- ✔ In cases of cyst–duct communication, stenosis or obstruction of the duct markedly increases the duration of drainage. Many prefer surgical or endoscopic drainage in these cases.
- ✔ For pancreatic abscesses, both percutaneous and endoscopic catheter drainage are viable options.
- ✘ Percutaneous drainage of sterile, acute fluid collections or simple pseudocysts should be avoided if possible because of the risk for superinfection.

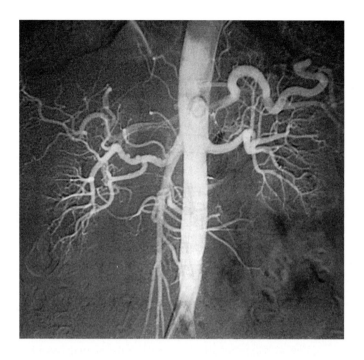

■ Clinical Presentation

A 42-year-old patient presents with hypertension refractory to medical management.

■ **Imaging Findings**

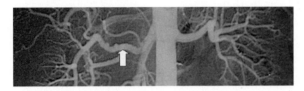

Conventional aortography shows beading of the right renal artery (*arrow*), indicating fibromuscular dysplasia (FMD).

■ **Differential Diagnosis**

- *Renal fibromuscular dysplasia (FMD):* Indicated by beading of the renal artery sparing the medial third.
- *Atherosclerosis:* Unlikely in a young adult with minimal arterial findings visible elsewhere.

■ **Essential Facts**

- FMD is a rare, noninflammatory disease of unknown etiology described in persons of all ages but most commonly in women (4:1) 30 to 50 years of age.
- Patients present with hypertension (FMD is the cause of 10% of cases of renovascular hypertension) and/or renal failure. Smoking accelerates the onset and increases the severity.
- Subtypes include intimal, medial (99% of cases of hypertension), and adventitial.
- Treatment is clinical observation for asymptomatic patients, angioplasty (first-line) for symptomatic patients, and surgery (aortorenal bypass) for patients with refractory cases. Unlike atherosclerosis, FMD rarely requires endovascular stent placement.

■ **Other Imaging Findings**

- Conventional angiography, computed tomographic angiography, and magnetic resonance angiography demonstrate beading of the renal artery that typically spares the medial third, is usually unilateral and right-sided, and occasionally involves branch vessels.
- Associated findings may include true and dissecting aneurysms, arteriovenous fistulas, thrombosis, and distal embolization.
- Other distributions affected may include the iliac, carotid, mesenteric, and brachial arteries.

✔ **Pearls & ✗ Pitfalls**

- ✔ Angioplasty results in high rates of technical success (> 90%), patency, and clinical response.
- ✔ The primary patency rate at 4 years is 69%.
- ✔ The cumulative patency rate at 4 years is 85 to 94%.
- ✔ Clinical response: for patients with hypertension, the cure rate is 22 to 39%, and the improvement rate is 31 to 59%.
- ✗ Complications include dissection, rupture, occlusion, and distal embolization with infarction.
- ✗ Complication rates for angioplasty of FMD are much lower than those for angioplasty of atherosclerotic renal arteries.
- ✗ Arterial irregularity may persist after angioplasty, but the clinical response is excellent, and the urge to overdilate should be resisted.

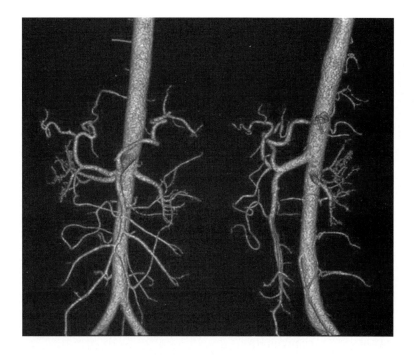

■ Clinical Presentation

The patient is a 57-year old man scheduled for chemoembolization of a hepatocellular carcinoma.

■ Imaging Findings

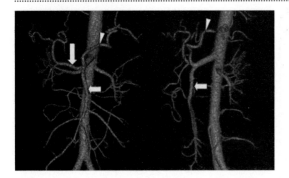

Three-dimensional volume-rendered computed tomographic angiogram (CTA) shows a common arterial trunk supplying the splenic (*arrowheads*), superior mesenteric (*small arrows*), and common hepatic (*large arrow*) arteries.

■ Differential Diagnosis

- *Celicomesenteric trunk:* Indicated by a common origin of the celiac artery and superior mesenteric artery (SMA).

■ Essential Facts

- Celicomesenteric trunk is a mesenteric arterial anomaly in which a common trunk supplies the origins of the celiac artery and the SMA. It occurs in < 1% of persons.
- Clinical significance: compared with persons who have separate origins of the celiac and mesenteric arteries, these patients are more prone to mesenteric ischemia if stenosis or obstruction develops in the trunk because of the larger distribution supplied by a single vessel.
- Mesenteric arterial anomalies deserve careful consideration because they can influence the severity of mesenteric ischemia and the clinical success and complication rates of procedures such as transarterial chemoembolization (TACE) of liver tumors and abdominal operations such as liver transplant.
- Other anomalies of the hepatic artery (HA) include the following:
  - Replaced right HA off SMA (< 16%)
  - Replaced left HA off left gastric artery (< 10%)
  - Replaced left and right HAs (< 1%)
  - Accessory left HA (< 8%)
  - Accessory right HA (< 7%)
  - Replaced common HA from SMA (< 5%)
  - Other (< 1%)

- Other HA branch anomalies include the following:
  - Right gastric: normal origin is proper HA, anomalous origin is gastroduodenal artery (GDA) or left, right, or common HA.
  - Cystic: normal origin is right HA, anomalous origin is replaced right, accessory right, common, or left HA.
  - Pancreaticoduodenal: normal origin is GDA, anomalous origin is HA branches.
  - Dorsal pancreatic: normal origin is splenic artery, anomalous origin is right HA.

■ Other Imaging Findings

- Anomalous mesenteric arteries can be detected with conventional angiography, CTA, or magnetic resonance angiography.

✔ Pearls & ✘ Pitfalls

- ✔ Injection of chemoembolization or radiotherapy agents into anomalous branches of the HA (nontarget embolization) can injure the corresponding organ.
- ✔ In many cases, nontarget chemoembolization of these anomalous arteries can be avoided by further subselection of HA branches to tumor, or by coil embolization of these anomalous vessels before the injection of chemotherapeutic agents.
- ✘ Chemoembolization of the stomach or duodenum can cause necrosis, ulceration, or perforation.
- ✘ Chemoembolization of the cystic artery can cause chemical cholecystitis.
- ✘ Chemoembolization of the dorsal pancreatic or pancreaticoduodenal artery can cause pancreatitis.

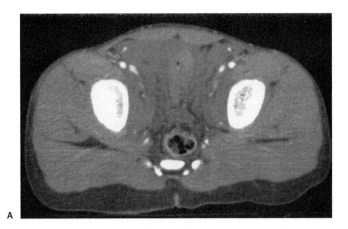

A

■ Clinical Presentation

A 7-year-old boy struck by a car is brought to the emergency department.

Further Work-up

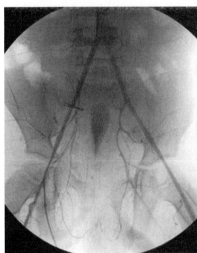

B

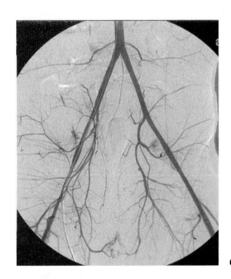

C

■ Imaging Findings

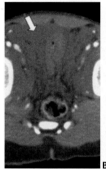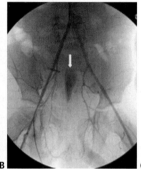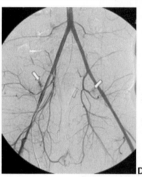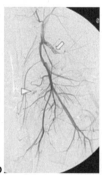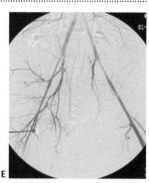

A   B   C   D   E

(A) Selected pelvic computed tomographic (CT) scan shows hematoma (*arrow*). **(B)** Selected pelvic angiogram shows teardrop-shaped bladder (*arrow*) compressed by hematoma. **(C)** Digital subtraction angiogram shows bilateral hemorrhage from the superior gluteal arteries (*arrows*). **(D)** Selected an-giogram of the left internal iliac artery after coil embolization of the superior gluteal artery (*arrow*) shows additional focus of hemorrhage (*arrowhead*). **(E)** Pelvic angiogram after Gelfoam embolization of both internal iliac arteries shows no further extravasation.

■ Differential Diagnosis

- ***Pelvic trauma***

■ Essential Facts

- High-energy blunt pelvic trauma requires rapid, multidisciplinary management to prevent death.
- The clinical presentation—stable or unstable—determines the outcome and treatment plan.
- Unstable patients (mortality > 40%) often undergo emergent exploratory surgery, but embolization may be attempted if timely.
- Stable patients (mortality < 5%) typically undergo CT and imaging work-up (see below), and treatment depends on the origin of pelvic hemorrhage—either venous or arterial.
- Venous bleeding is most common and usually responds to external fixation with application of a pelvic binder, antishock trousers, or a C-clamp.
- Arterial bleeding, which occurs in 10 to 20% of patients, is the leading associated cause of death and is best treated with embolization.
- Embolization is usually performed with Gelfoam, coils, or a combination of these.
- Surgery is risky in trauma patients because the abdominal tamponade resulting from the tense hematoma is released by laparotomy.
- Anterior pelvic bleeding is often from the internal pudendal or obturator artery.
- Posterior pelvic bleeding is often from the superior gluteal or lateral sacral artery. Posterior element disruption is a major risk factor for arterial injury. The superior gluteal artery is the most commonly transected vessel.
- Types of injury may include vasospasm, transection, pseudoaneurysm, and arteriovenous fistula.

■ Other Imaging Finding

- Diagnostic imaging work-up for pelvic trauma usually involves portable radiography of the chest, abdomen, and pelvis, focused abdominal ultrasound, and CT.

✔ Pearls & ✘ Pitfalls

- ✔ Angiography and embolization for pelvic trauma is carried out by catheterizing the common femoral artery opposite the side of injury.
- ✔ Multifocal bleeding is often embolized by injecting Gelfoam slurry proximally in the internal iliac artery to occlude multiple arterial distributions. Bilateral internal iliac artery embolization may be necessary.
- ✔ Focal sites of bleeding may be successfully treated with more selective coil embolization.
- ✔ Unstable patients should be treated quickly, and more proximal (internal iliac artery) embolization with coils and Gelfoam may be preferable to time-consuming subselective embolization in some cases.
- ✘ Complications of pelvic embolization include nontarget embolization, complications at the access site, and rarely impotence. Impotence may be due to urologic and lumbosacral plexus injuries rather than arterial insufficiency caused by embolization.
- ✘ Bladder or rectal ischemia due to bilateral occlusion of the internal iliac arteries is exceedingly rare and often absent in large studies.
- ✘ Arteries that are not visualized may be transected, in vasospasm, or thrombosed.
- ✘ Transected arteries can cause delayed catastrophic hemorrhage as vasospasm subsides.

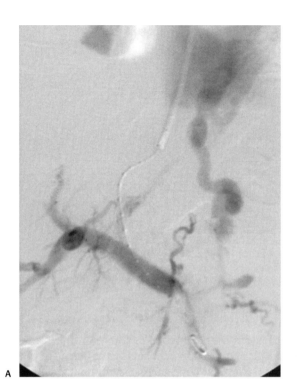

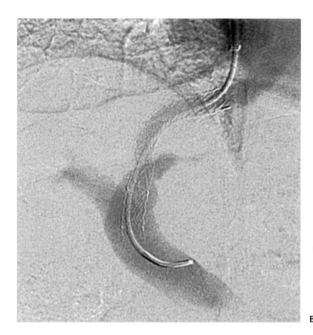

A

B

Clinical Presentation

A 51-year-old man presents with obtundation after a transjugular intrahepatic portosystemic shunt (TIPS) procedure.

■ Imaging Findings

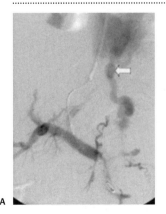
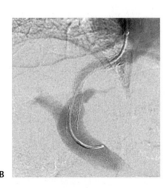
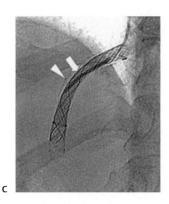

(A) Transjugular portal venogram shows a large gastroesophageal varix (*arrow*). (B) TIPS placed. (C) TIPS reduction by deployment of a constrained covered stent (*arrow*) within the preexisting TIPS stent (*arrowhead*).

■ Differential Diagnosis

• **_Hepatic encephalopathy after TIPS placement_**

■ Essential Facts

• TIPS-related hepatic encephalopathy is believed to result when nitrogenous products from the intestine, such as ammonia, bypass hepatic filtration and enter the intracranial circulation.
• The clinical presentation includes obtundation, disorientation, and confusion.
• The incidence of hepatic encephalopathy after TIPS placement is ~20%.
• Predisposing factors include a diet high in protein, diuresis, sepsis, use of sedatives, hypokalemia, dehydration, and preexisting hepatic dysfunction.
• Medical treatment should be attempted first—including a protein-restricted, high-fiber diet, nonabsorbable disaccharides such as oral or rectal lactulose, oral nonabsorbable antibiotics such as neomycin, and colonic cleansing with mannitol solution or laxatives. Approximately 5% cases are refractory, and endovascular treatment is necessary.
• Endovascular treatment options include use of a constricted, covered stent to reduce the diameter of the TIPS, coil embolization of physiologic portosystemic shunts, and coil embolization of the TIPS.
• Surgical treatment usually involves a liver transplant and is reserved for severe cases.

■ Other Imaging Findings

• With the appropriate clinical presentation after TIPS placement, hepatic encephalopathy should be considered regardless of the imaging appearance and ultrasonographic features of the TIPS.

✔ Pearls & ✘ Pitfalls

✔ Endovascular reduction of a TIPS may be accomplished by two basic methods:
✔ A new covered stent, constricted in the middle by a loop of suture, is deployed within the preexisting TIPS.
✔ Two new stents, parallel to each other, are deployed within the preexisting TIPS, one a covered self-expanding stent and the other an uncovered balloon-expandable stent that is shorter than the self-expanding stent. The short balloon-expandable stent narrows the lumen of the self-expanding stent.
✘ Recurrent variceal bleeding after placement of a constricted stent for encephalopathy may necessitate balloon dilation of the constricted stent. Recurrent variceal bleeding after coil embolization of a TIPS may necessitate placement of a new TIPS.
✘ Nontarget embolization of coils during TIPS occlusion results in embolization of a pulmonary arterial branch.
✘ Death due to severe decrease in cardiac output, metabolic acidosis, and hypotension has been reported (extremely rare) as a consequence of abrupt shunt occlusion.

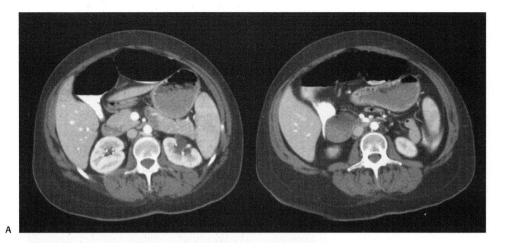

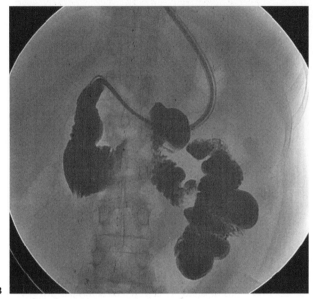

Clinical Presentation

A 25-year-old patient presents with midepigastric pain, vomiting, and weight loss.

■ Imaging Findings

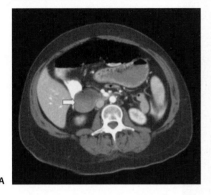
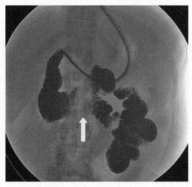

A

B

DISCOVERY LIBRARY
LEVEL 5 SWCC
DERRIFORD HOSPITAL
DERRIFORD ROAD
PLYMOUTH
PL6 8DH

(A) Infused computed tomographic (CT) scan shows dilatation of the second portion of the duodenum (*arrow*) with constriction of the third portion between the superior mesenteric artery (SMA) and the aorta. **(B)** Upper gastrointestinal (GI) barium study shows dilatation of the first and second portion of the duodenum with vertical bandlike constriction (*arrow*) of the third portion over the spine.

■ Differential Diagnosis

- *Superior mesenteric artery syndrome:* Indicated by dilatation of the second portion and vertical compression of the third portion of the duodenum as it passes behind the SMA.
- Congenital or acquired entities such as intestinal pseudo-obstruction or diabetes can result in duodenal obstruction, but typically without the focal narrowing noted in this case.
- Malignancies intrinsic or extrinsic to the duodenum can result in focal narrowing, but no masses are detected by CT in this case.

■ Essential Facts

- Partial or complete obstruction of the third portion of the duodenum due to constriction between the aorta and SMA, also called *cast syndrome*, can occur in both children and adults, but most patients range in age from 10 to 30 years.
- The incidence is < 1%.
- The presentation includes symptoms of upper GI obstruction—vomiting (often bilious), midepigastric pain, and early satiety. Symptoms are increased in the supine position.
- Predisposing factors include low weight-to-height ratio, low origin of the SMA, high position of the ligament of Treitz, and any condition that narrows the angle between the SMA and the aorta from the normal 45 degrees to < 25 degrees, including the following: scoliosis, lumbar lordosis, previous spine surgery, Harrington rods, spica casts, and marked weight loss with depletion of mesenteric fat.

- Medical treatment is first-line, including the following: placement of a nasogastric tube for initial decompression, placement of a nasojejunal tube for feeding (a dual-lumen tube accomplishes both), parenteral nutrition if necessary, and gradual advancement to oral liquids and soft solids.
- Surgical treatment is indicated for refractory cases: open duodenojejunostomy or laparoscopic release of the ligament of Treitz.
- Upper GI barium study shows vertical constriction of the third portion of duodenum, delayed emptying across the obstruction, antiperistaltic waves, and a normal mucosal fold pattern.
- CT scan or abdominal ultrasonogram may show a reduced angle and distance (< 9 mm) between the aorta and SMA.

✔ Pearls & ✘ Pitfalls

- ✔ Some experts think that SMA syndrome is overdiagnosed.
- ✔ A complete work-up for other causes of upper GI obstruction should be performed, including upper GI endoscopy.
- ✘ Failure to diagnose and correct SMA syndrome can lead to associated peptic ulcer disease, malnutrition, and further weight loss.

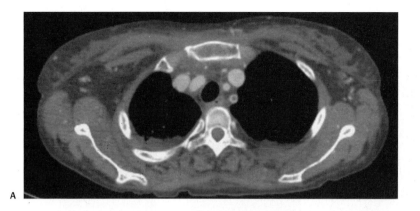

A

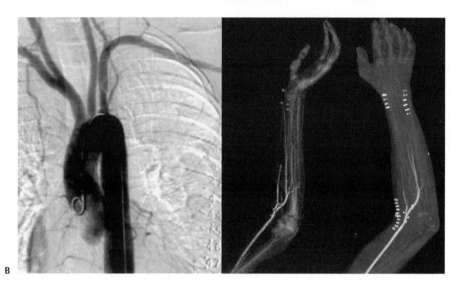

B

■ Clinical Presentation

A 35-year-old man presents to the emergency department with an abrupt onset of pain and pallor in the left arm.

■ Imaging Findings

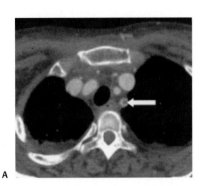
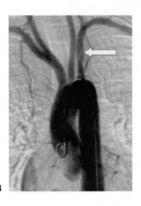
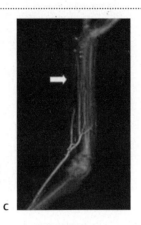
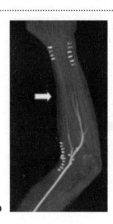

A   B   C   D

(A) Infused computed tomographic (CT) scan shows filling defect within the proximal portion of the left subclavian artery (*arrow*). **(B)** Angiogram of the aortic arch shows subclavian artery filling defect proximal to the takeoff of the vertebral artery (*arrow*). **(C,D)** Three-dimensional volume-rendered and maximal-intensity-projection images from a computed tomographic angiogram (CTA) of the left arm show abrupt occlusion of the forearm trifurcation arteries, indicating distal thromboembolism (*arrows*). Surgical clips indicate attempted surgical revascularization.

■ Differential Diagnosis

- **Subclavian artery thrombosis with distal thromboembolism:** Indicated by the symptoms, the acute presentation, and the imaging findings of an acute arterial filling defect and distal abrupt occlusions.

■ Essential Facts

- The presentation varies with the acuteness and severity and may include acute ischemia after a long history of arm claudication. Look for a cold, pale, or cyanotic arm with reduced or absent pulses and/or gangrene.
- Thrombosis and marked underlying atherosclerosis may result in a milder presentation because of the previous recruitment of collateral pathways. Thrombosis and lack of underlying atherosclerosis may result in severe limb ischemia.
- Predisposing factors include the following: right-to-left shunts (paradoxical embolus), repetitive athletic or occupational trauma, thoracic outlet syndrome (TOS), atherosclerosis, subclavian catheterization, aneurysms, and hypercoagulable states.
- The medical work-up should include a search for hypercoagulable states.
- TOS can injure the subclavian artery as it passes through a narrowed thoracic outlet between the clavicle and first rib during hyperabduction. TOS can cause thrombosis, stenosis, aneurysm, or dissection.
- Surgical thrombectomy of an acute subclavian artery thrombus is often the first-line treatment because catheter manipulation can result in vertebral artery thromboembolism. TOS is treated with release of the anterior scalene muscle and resection of the first rib. Chronic atherosclerosis may require bypass.

- Endovascular treatment may be first-line in some cases (e.g., thrombolysis of acute thromboembolism distal to the vertebral artery or angioplasty/stent placement for chronic occlusions).
- Angiography (conventional, magnetic resonance, CT) should include the aortic arch and the entire extremity. Conventional angiography should include two views of the thoracic arch and great vessels.
- Thromboembolism in the distal part of the arm without visible proximal arterial pathology may be caused by TOS. An angiogram of the aortic arch in the hyperabducted (stressed) position should be obtained.
- CT or chest radiography may demonstrate underlying bony causes, including cervical ribs, congenital or post-traumatic deformity, and exophytic tumors such as benign exostoses.

■ Other Imaging Finding

- Echocardiography should be performed to evaluate for a possible cardiac source of subclavian thrombus.

✔ Pearls & ✘ Pitfalls

- ✔ Subclavian steal syndrome describes reversal of flow direction within the ipsilateral vertebral artery to supply the subclavian artery distal to the point of obstruction. It presents with vertigo and dizziness.
- ✔ Thrombolysis of acute thrombus of the proximal subclavian artery has been described, but surgical thrombectomy is typically preferred to avoid the complication of stroke associated with catheter manipulation.
- ✘ Posterior cerebral thromboembolism may result from catheter manipulation of acute thrombus in the proximal portion of the subclavian artery.
- ✘ Chylothorax may result from injury of the thoracic duct during surgical repair.

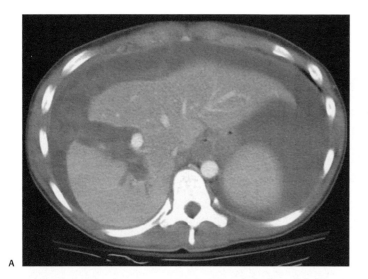

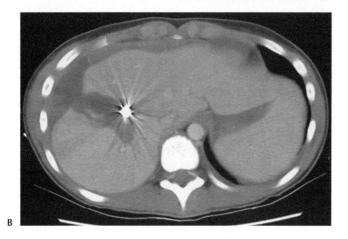

■ Clinical Presentation

A 16-year-old girl is brought to the emergency department after a skiing accident. She is hypotensive and tachycardic.

■ Imaging Findings

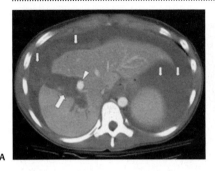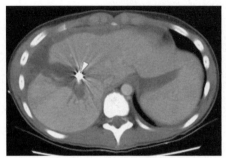

A   B

(A) Contrast-enhanced computed tomographic (CT) scan shows a grade 5 liver laceration (*large arrow*), a hepatic artery pseudoaneurysm (*arrowhead*), and acute blood in the perihepatic and perisplenic spaces (*small arrows*). (B) Contrast-enhanced CT scan shows successful coil embolization of the pseudoaneurysm (*arrowhead*).

■ Differential Diagnosis

• *Traumatic hepatic laceration*

■ Essential Facts

• Traumatic hepatic laceration occurs during blunt injury to the abdomen. It is graded as follows:
  1. Parenchymal depth < 1 cm
  2. Parenchymal depth 1 to 3 cm
  3. Parenchymal depth > 3 cm
  4. Involvement of 25 to 75% of a hepatic lobe or of 1 to 3 Couinaud segments within a single lobe
  5. Involvement of > 75% of a hepatic lobe or of > 3 Couinaud segments within a single lobe and/or juxtahepatic venous injuries (retrohepatic caval or hepatic venous avulsion)
  6. Hepatic avulsion
• The clinical presentation determines the work-up. Stable patients go to contrast-enhanced CT, and unstable patients often go to exploratory laparotomy.
• The treatment depends on the presentation and findings and may be medical management, transarterial embolization (TAE), or exploratory laparotomy.
• Medical management involves the intravenous administration of fluids, blood products, and vasopressors.
• TAE is considered a first-line treatment in stable patients with evidence of continued blood loss despite medical management and in patients with active extravasation or an arterial defect such as a pseudoaneurysm. After successful TAE, surgery is usually unnecessary.
• Exploratory laparotomy is reserved for patients whose condition is refractory to TAE and for patients presenting with profound hypotension refractory to fluid resuscitation.
• Contrast-enhanced CT shows the degree of hepatic laceration, associated injuries, the extent of bleeding, active extravasation, and occasionally the exact vessel injured.

■ Other Imaging Finding

• Conventional angiography is performed with the intent to embolize and may show active extravasation, pseudoaneurysm, arterial transection or dissection, or arterial spasm or thrombosis.

✔ Pearls & ✗ Pitfalls

✔ The embolic agent used for TAE in these cases varies with the underlying injury.
✔ Diffuse bleeding resulting from a high-grade liver laceration is often treated by injection of large-sized particles (Gelfoam, polyvinyl alcohol, or tris-acryl gel spheres) into multiple arterial distributions.
✔ Focal sources of bleeding, such as arteriovenous fistulas and pseudoaneurysms, are usually treated with coil embolization.
✔ Injury to a large arterial branch may be treated with coils, a combination of coils and Gelfoam, or placement of a covered stent.
✗ Complications of TAE are uncommon and include necrosis, abscess formation, nontarget embolization, catheter-related arterial injury, and access site injury. Oxygen supply from the portal system minimizes the risk for necrosis.
✗ Profound hypotension may indicate bleeding from a source not amenable to TAE, such as a ruptured or avulsed inferior vena cava, hepatic vein, or portal vein. Repair with a covered stent has been described, but emergent exploratory laparotomy is usually indicated.
✗ Laparotomy for hepatic laceration involves the sudden release of the protective effects of abdominal tamponade, placing patients at risk for death. In addition, surgery may require the resection of large amounts of normal tissue.

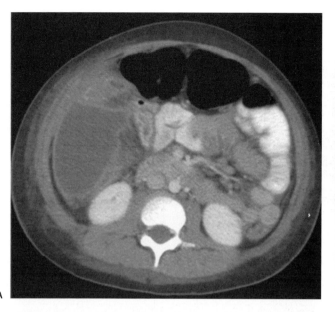

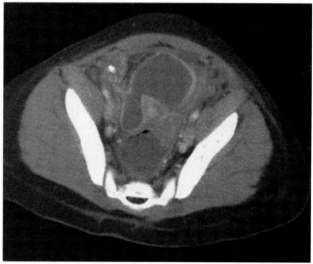

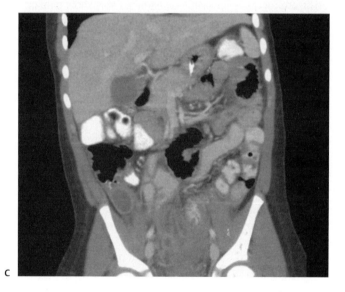

■ Clinical Presentation

A 28-year-old man presents with fever 10 days after the onset of abdominal pain.

■ Imaging Findings

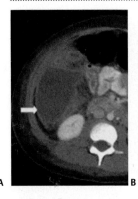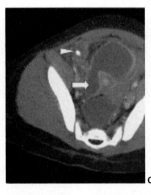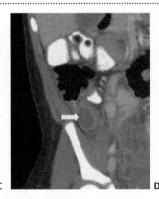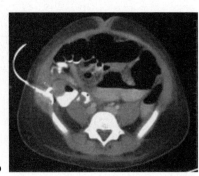

A   B   C   D

(A) Contrast-enhanced computed tomographic (CT) scan shows a walled-off fluid collection (*arrow*). **(B)** Second component of the fluid collection (*arrow*) and a calcification suspected to be an appendicolith (*arrowhead*).

(C) Coronal reformatting shows infracecal location of the collection (*arrow*). **(D)** Image obtained after drain placement.

■ Differential Diagnosis

- **Appendiceal abscess:** Is most likely given the probable appendicolith and right lower quadrant fluid component.
- *Diverticular abscess:* May be indistinguishable but more commonly occurs on the left.

■ Essential Facts

- Appendicitis results from luminal obstruction and occurs in 7% of the population at any age (most commonly 10–30 years). Appendiceal abscess results from the rupture of an inflamed appendix.
- Predisposing conditions include a diet low in fiber and a familial tendency.
- Symptoms of appendicitis may progress over 1 to 2 days from early, diffuse midepigastric pain to delayed, focal right lower quadrant pain. Variations in the position of the appendix cause marked variability in the presentation.
- Contrast-enhanced CT may show an additional finding of lack of contrast filling to the bulbous tip.
- Treatment varies according to the presentation and may be medical management, percutaneous catheter drainage (PCD), or surgery.
- Appendectomy by either open laparotomy or laparoscopy is required in cases of acute appendicitis associated with peritoneal signs.
- PCD is an option for patients with a mature (walled-off) abscess and no peritoneal signs. Surgery is not required in up to 80% of such cases. In the remainder, surgery is delayed to allow systemic infection to resolve so that a cleaner, more elective procedure is possible—so-called interval appendectomy.
- Medical management without surgery or PCD may be successful in patients with small (< 3 cm) abscesses that respond to antibiotics.

■ Other Imaging Finding

- Ultrasonography for acute appendicitis may show pain on compression, an outer diameter > 6 mm, lack of compressibility and peristalsis, and adjacent fluid.

✔ Pearls & ✘ Pitfalls

- ✔ For patients with appendicitis, mature abscesses may be treated with an initial combination of PCD, antibiotics, bowel rest, and hyperalimentation.
- ✔ For patients with Crohn's disease, mature abscesses may be treated with the same regimen plus high-dose steroids for a period before surgery.
- ✔ Drain management is as follows:
  1. Drain removal is possible after resolution of fever (usually within 48 hours), normalization of leukocytosis (usually within 5 days), and reduction of drain output to < 20 mL/d.
  2. Catheter clogging is indicated by a sudden cessation of output, leakage of pus around the catheter at the skin, and resumption of fever and leukocytosis. Exchange/upsizing is indicated.
- ✘ Complications of PCD of abdominal abscesses include nontarget catheterization (e.g., colon), abscess-to-enteric fistula formation, cross-contamination of sterile spaces, and systemic spread of infection (sepsis).
- ✘ For inadvertent catheterization of the colon, allow time (4 weeks) for tract maturation, which can be verified by over-the-wire tractogram, before tube removal.

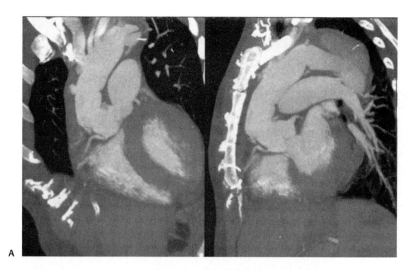

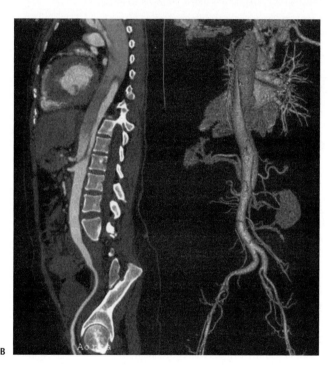

A

B

■ Clinical Presentation

A 49-year-old woman has a history of ascending aortic aneurysm repair.

■ Imaging Findings

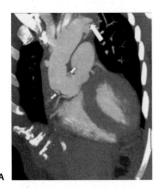
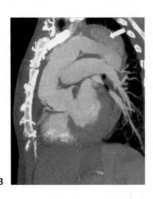
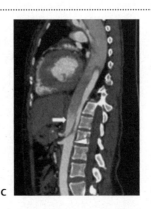
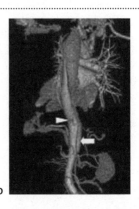

A   B   C   D

(A) Oblique, coronal reformatting of a contrast-enhanced (CT) scan shows a linear aortic filling defect (*large arrow*) distal to the left subclavian artery (*small arrows,* tube graft). **(B)** Oblique, sagittal reformatting shows contrast within the false lumen of a Stanford type B aortic dissection (*arrow*). **(C)** Sagittal reformatting shows supply to the celiac artery by the false lumen (*arrow*) and supply to the superior mesenteric artery by the true lumen (*arrowhead*). **(D)** Three-dimensional volume-rendered posterior image shows the renal arteries filling from the true lumen, just below the lowest point of dissection (*arrowhead,* true lumen; *arrow,* false lumen).

■ Differential Diagnosis

• ***Dissecting aortic aneurysm, Stanford type B***

■ Essential Facts

• This is a tear in the intima of the aorta with dissection of blood into the media.
• Locations are descending only, 50%; ascending or ascending plus descending, 50%.
• The presentation is typically ripping chest pain but varies with the location and involvement of the great vessels, aortic valve, pericardial sac, and coronary arteries.
• Risk factors include the following: atherosclerotic disease, trauma, bicuspid aortic valve, coarctation, pregnancy, cocaine use, cystic medial necrosis, some connective tissue diseases (Marfan syndrome, Ehlers–Danlos syndrome), and homocystinuria.
• Mortality rate is ~1%/h for the first 48 hours.
• Stanford classification
  • Type A: ascending aorta
  • Type B: distal to origin of subclavian artery
• DeBakey classification
  • Type 1: ascending aorta, aortic arch, descending aorta
  • Type 2: limited to ascending aorta
  • Type 3: limited to descending aorta distal to origin of left subclavian artery
• Type A is treated surgically to prevent propagation to the aortic root with rupture, pericardial tamponade, or involvement of the coronary arteries. Type B is usually treated medically unless there is rupture, uncontrolled hypertension, or organ ischemia.
• CT/CT angiography (CTA) offers the best anatomic delineation of aortic dissection from the arch to the pelvis and accurately shows dissection flaps, true and false lumina, organ perfusion, and complications (rupture).
• Medical treatment is with antihypertensives and analgesics.

• Surgical treatment is with fenestration (see Pearls) and primary repair.
• Endovascular treatment is with stent-grafts, stents, fenestration, or some combination.

■ Other Imaging Findings

• CT/CTA, magnetic resonance imaging/magnetic resonance angiography, and transesophageal echocardiography (TEE) have similar diagnostic yields with high rates of sensitivity and specificity for aortic dissection.
• Conventional angiography provides an excellent demonstration of branch vessel perfusion by a true or false lumen and is reserved for surgical planning and for the evaluation and treatment of complications.
• TEE allows a fast bedside examination of unstable patients and may show type B entry/reentry sites not visible on CTA, in addition to type A coronary involvement, pericardial effusion, and aortic regurgitation.

✔ Pearls & ✘ Pitfalls

✔ Cystic medial necrosis occurs with aging and connective tissue diseases like Marfan syndrome. The breakdown of smooth muscle and connective tissue in the media predisposes patients to dissection.
✔ Fenestration is puncturing across the intimal flap, which creates a rent between the false and true lumina.
✔ Stents can be used to tack down the intimal flap or revascularize compromised branch vessels.
✔ Stent-grafts have been used to seal the proximal entry point of the flap.
✘ Risks of stents and stent-grafts include stent migration, continued organ ischemia or infarction (particularly mesenteric, renal), and paralysis due to inadvertent obstruction of a spinal artery.

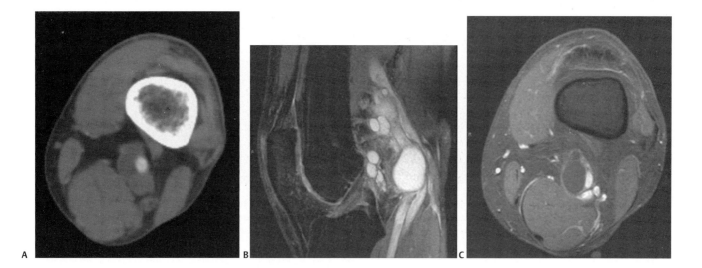

A

B

C

◼ Clinical Presentation

A 45-year-old nonsmoker presents with rapidly progressing unilateral, intermittent claudication. On physical examination, a loss of the distal pulses is noted during knee flexion.

■ Imaging Findings

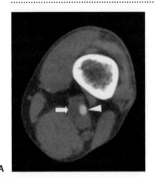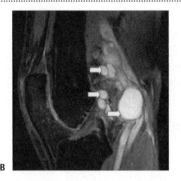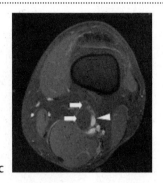

A   B   C

(A) Axial contrast-enhanced computed tomographic (CT) scan shows nonenhancing structure (*arrow*) adjacent to the popliteal artery (*arrowhead*). **(B)** Sagittal, proton density, fat saturation magnetic resonance image (MRI) shows ovoid, hyperintense structures (*arrows*) in the popliteal fossa. **(C)** Axial, fast spoiled gradient echo MRI shows ovoid structures with low signal intensity (*arrows*) partially compressing the popliteal artery (*arrowhead*).

■ Differential Diagnosis

- ***Cystic adventitial disease (CAD):*** Is indicated by multiple cysts in the popliteal fossa with appropriate imaging characteristics.

■ Essential Facts

- CAD is a rare vascular disorder in which intramural mucinous cysts rich in amino acids expand and compress the vascular lumen. It tends to occur in young to middle-aged men.
- The location is usually arterial, but venous cases have been reported. CAD is usually popliteal and unilateral, but it has been reported in the external iliac and common femoral arteries as well as the brachial, radial, and ulnar arteries.
- The presentation of popliteal CAD is related to the morphology of the disease. Luminal narrowing due to compression by cysts can cause rapidly progressing claudication; superimposed thrombosis can cause acute ischemia.
- The pathogenesis is theorized to be either developmental, with ectopic mucin-secreting synovial cells in the adventitia, or traumatic, with expansile cystic necrosis.
- The prognosis is typically progression to claudication or ischemia unless treated. Rare spontaneous regression has been described.
- The treatment is either surgical or endovascular.
- Surgical treatment is definitive, including some combination of cyst aspiration or evacuation, arterial patching, and/or arterial resection with bypass.

- Endovascular treatment has been reported and is limited to stent or stent-graft placement. Angioplasty alone has not been successful.
- CT/CT angiography shows an arterial lumen compressed by low-density intramural structures.
- MRI/MR angiography shows cysts to be low-intensity on T1-weighted and high-intensity on T2-weighted images. Imaging is typically performed with fat saturation.

■ Other Imaging Findings

- Doppler ultrasound may demonstrate the cysts and compression of the popliteal artery, and it may help distinguish CAD from Baker's cysts and aneurysms/pseudoaneurysms.
- Conventional angiography typically shows focal luminal narrowing caused by extrinsic compression.

✔ Pearls & ✘ Pitfalls

- ✔ Popliteal artery disease in a young to middle-aged adult may be caused by CAD, popliteal entrapment syndrome, popliteal artery aneurysms, trauma (dissection, pseudoaneurysm, or thrombosis), or accelerated atherosclerosis.
- ✔ CAD may be distinguished on physical examination by the loss of distal pulses during knee flexion resulting from pronounced arterial compression by adjacent cysts.
- ✘ Structures adjacent to the popliteal artery on cross-sectional imaging may include thrombosed aneurysms/ pseudoaneurysms, thrombosed varicose veins, Baker's cysts, and soft-tissue tumors, in addition to CAD.

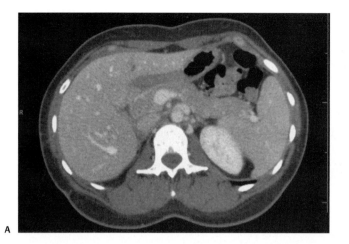

A

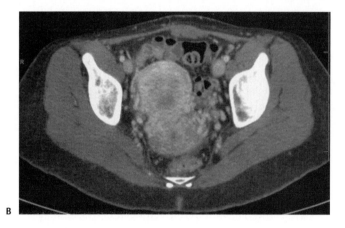

B

▣ Clinical Presentation

A 37-year-old woman presents with chronic pelvic pain and hematuria.

■ Imaging Findings

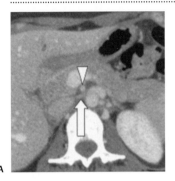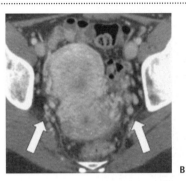

(A) Contrast-enhanced computed tomographic (CT) scan shows compression of the left renal vein (*arrow*) as it passes behind the superior mesenteric artery (SMA: *arrowhead*). (B) Pelvic image shows multiple dilated veins on both sides (*arrows*).

■ Differential Diagnosis

- **Nutcracker syndrome (NS):** Indicated by the symptoms and constriction of the left renal vein by the SMA.
- *Pelvic congestion syndrome (PCS):* Secondary to incompetent ovarian vein produces identical pelvic findings without renal vein obstruction.

■ Essential Facts

- NS is compression of the left renal vein between the SMA and the aorta that causes increased pressure in the renal vein and dilatation of the gonadal and pelvic veins.
- NS usually presents in thin, younger women but has been described in children. Symptoms may include gross hematuria, proteinuria, and/or pelvic congestion syndrome (see Pearls).
- Recent weight loss is a risk factor.
- Endovascular stent placement in the left renal vein has been reported, but its utility is controversial.
- Contrast-enhanced CT may show extrinsic compression of the renal vein between the SMA and aorta, dilated pelvic veins, and the absence of alternative pelvic pathology to explain the patient's symptoms.

■ Other Imaging Findings

- Conventional venography is the diagnostic imaging tool of choice and typically shows compression of the left renal vein, perirenal varices, retrograde filling of a dilated left gonadal vein (> 5 mm), and an elevated pressure gradient between the renal vein and inferior vena cava (> 2 mm Hg).

✔ Pearls & ✘ Pitfalls

- ✔ PCS is chronic pelvic pain in the setting of dilated ovarian (left > right) and periuterine veins and/or dyspareunia, labial and perineal varices, and the absence of an alternative explanation such as endometriosis, fibroids, adenomyosis, or pelvic infection.
- ✔ Ultrasound, magnetic resonance imaging, and conventional venography should be performed with the patient upright or in the reverse Trendelenburg position if possible because imaging in the supine position can underestimate the degree of gonadal and pelvic venous dilatation in cases of PCS.
- ✘ The effectiveness of stent placement to treat NS has not yet been established by prospective studies.
- ✘ Most cases of PCS occur in the absence of NS and are caused by retrograde reflux of blood from the renal veins through the gonadal veins into the pelvic veins as a consequence of valvular incompetence.
- ✘ In cases of PCS without NS, gonadal vein embolization (with coils or sclerosant agents), laparoscopic gonadal vein ligation, and hysterectomy are treatment options.

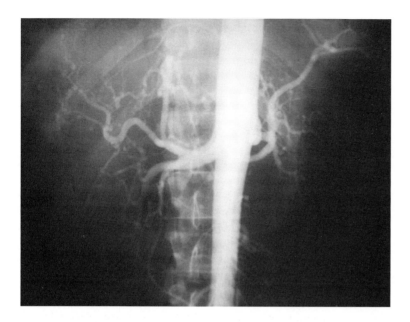

Clinical Presentation

A 54-year-old man presents with fever, abdominal pain, weight loss, and malaise.

■ Imaging Findings

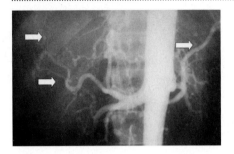

Conventional aortogram shows innumerable small aneurysms involving branches of the hepatic, splenic, and mesenteric arteries (*arrows*).

■ Differential Diagnosis

- *Polyarteritis nodosa (PAN)*
- For multiple microaneurysms of the visceral arteries, include other vasculitides, such as *systemic lupus erythematosus* and *Wegener's granulomatosis,* as well as *amphetamine abuse* ("speed kidney").

■ Essential Facts

- PAN is a necrotizing vasculitis of unknown etiology affecting small and medium-sized arteries. It is most common in men (the male-to-female ratio is 2:1) in the 5th to 7th decades.
- It may affect any small to medium-sized arteries, including the renal (most commonly), hepatic, splenic, mesenteric, and skeletal arteries.
- PAN is diagnosed if any three of the following are present: weight loss ≥ 4 kg, livedo reticularis, testicular tenderness, myalgias, weakness or tenderness, neuropathy, diastolic blood pressure > 90 mm Hg, elevated blood urea nitrogen or creatinine level, hepatitis B, arteriographic abnormality, biopsy specimen of small or medium-sized artery containing polymorphonuclear leukocytes.
- Angiography may show occlusive lesions (most commonly), ectasia, and aneurysms, classically at branch points, ranging from microaneurysmal to 2 cm in diameter.

- The pathogenesis is arterial inflammation believed to be the sequela of immune complex deposition.
- Medical treatment is high-dose steroids and cytotoxic drugs.
- Endovascular treatment is limited to embolization of associated aneurysms and hemorrhage.

■ Other Imaging Findings

- Computed tomography (CT)/CT angiography is a common screening tool and may identify ischemia of the viscera or solid organs, in addition to larger aneurysms, bony lesions, or pulmonary involvement.
- Magnetic resonance imaging (MRI)/MR angiography may serve as an alternative screening tool, showing mucosal inflammation and granulomas in the paranasal sinuses.
- Conventional angiography remains the gold standard vascular study and is the best modality to demonstrate distal arterial microaneurysms.

✔ Pearls & ✘ Pitfalls

- ✔ The prognosis with treatment is relapse in 40% and 5-year survival of 80%. Without treatment, most patients die within 5 years.
- ✘ In patients who have PAN with an arterial abnormality, multiple aneurysms and microaneurysms are the classic finding but occur in only 60%. The nonspecific finding of occlusive lesions occurs in almost all such cases.

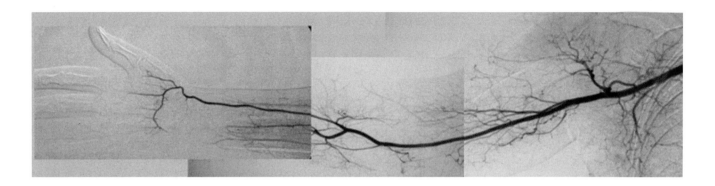

■ **Clinical Presentation**

A 53-year-old woman with rheumatoid arthritis presents with "cold" fingers.

■ Imaging Findings

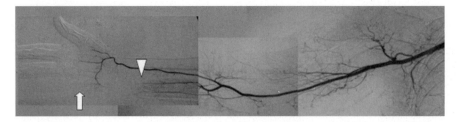

Conventional upper extremity angiogram shows absence of flow in all digital arteries (*arrow*) and abrupt termination of flow in the ulnar and interosseus arteries (*arrowhead*). The brachial and axillary arteries and branches appear normal. The next step would be intra-arterial administration of a vasodilator.

■ Differential Diagnosis

- **Secondary Raynaud's (Raynaud's phenomenon):** Suggested by the diffusely pruned small and medium-sized arteries and the history of rheumatoid arthritis.
- *Hypothenar hammer syndrome:* A possibility given the involvement of the ulnar artery, but diffuse digital arterial occlusion is not characteristic.
- *Embolic phenomenon:* A possibility given the relative lack of more proximal atherosclerotic disease and the diffuse occlusion of the distal small and medium-sized arteries.

■ Essential Facts

- Raynaud's is reversible diminished distal perfusion caused by vasospasm of the arterioles. Raynaud's phenomenon and Raynaud's disease are separate entities.
- The clinical presentation ranges from pallor to cyanosis, numbness, and pain, typically brought on by factors such as cold and stress.
- The risk is increased by alcohol and tobacco use.
- Raynaud's phenomenon, or secondary Raynaud's, is vasospasm superimposed on another disorder—most commonly scleroderma and mixed connective tissue disease, and less commonly a broad list of causes (autoimmune, infectious, neoplastic, metabolic, hematologic, pharmacologic, and environmental).
- Raynaud's disease, or primary Raynaud's, is vasospasm without an underlying disorder. The prevalence is 4 to 5% of the general population. It typically presents in the 2nd or 3rd decade and rarely causes tissue loss. The prognosis is good.

- The diagnosis is made by a careful history and physical examination. Imaging studies can be supportive in equivocal cases.
- Treatment options include surgical sympathectomy, vasodilators such as calcium channel blockers and prostaglandins, and the treatment of any underlying disorder (in secondary Raynaud's).
- Conventional angiography is typically performed before and after the injection of a vasodilator such as papaverine to determine the extent of reversible vasospasm versus fixed obstruction.

■ Other Imaging Findings

- For the diagnosis of Raynaud's, cold challenge testing with nuclear medicine technetium 99m scans (DTPA [diethylenetriamine penta-acetic acid] or sestamibi) or dynamic thermal imaging has been advocated.
- For all patients who have Raynaud's, suspected underlying disorders should be investigated with the appropriate imaging tests.

✔ Pearls & ✘ Pitfalls

- ✔ Environmental associations with Raynaud's phenomenon include frostbite and occupational exposure to vibrating tools or polyvinyl chloride.
- ✘ No imaging or laboratory test reliably confirms the diagnosis of Raynaud's disease. Clinical evaluation is critical.
- ✘ Any patient with the appropriate presentation should undergo a thorough evaluation for an underlying disorder before the clinician settles on the diagnosis of primary Raynaud's (Raynaud's disease).

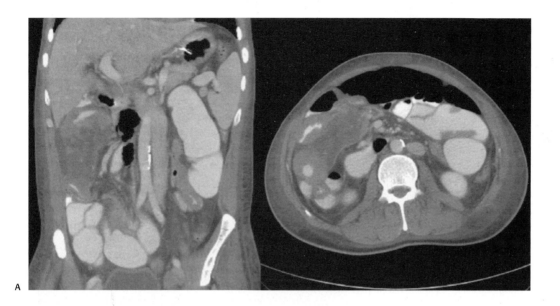

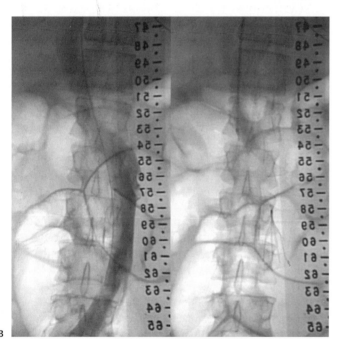

■ Clinical Presentation

A 46-year-old man with deep venous thrombosis (DVT) is scheduled for surgical resection of tumor in his right leg, pelvis, and abdomen.

■ Imaging Findings

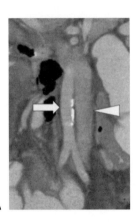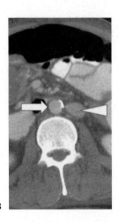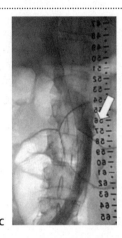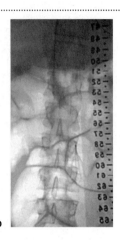

A B C D

(A,B) Coronal and axial contrast-enhanced computed tomographic (CT) images show transposition of the calcified aorta (*arrow*) and the inferior vena cava (IVC: *arrowhead*). **(C,D)** Venogram and fluoroscopic image after placement of a Tulip filter (Cook Medical, Bloomington, IN). The left-sided IVC drains into the left renal vein (*arrow*).

■ Differential Diagnosis

• **Transposition of the IVC**

■ Essential Facts

• An aberrant position of the IVC is to the left of the aorta and spine (prevalence < 0.5%).
• Both common iliac veins drain into a single left-sided IVC.
• The IVC ascends to the left of the aorta and spine to join the left renal vein.
• The left renal vein then crosses to the right side at its expected location between the aorta and superior mesenteric artery.
• The right renal vein joins the IVC below its junction with the left renal vein.

■ Other Imaging Finding

• Magnetic resonance imaging and CT can detect anomalies of the IVC and renal vein with sufficient sensitivity for planning surgical and radiologic procedures.

✔ Pearls & ✘ Pitfalls

✔ Other anomalies of the IVC and renal veins include circumaortic left renal vein, retroaortic left renal vein, multiple left or right renal veins, duplication of the IVC, azygos continuation of the IVC, and congenital megacava.
✔ Duplication of the IVC describes drainage of the right common iliac and renal veins into a right-sided IVC and drainage of the left common iliac and renal veins into a left-sided IVC. For adequate caval filtration, filters must be placed in each infrarenal IVC, or a single filter may be placed in the suprarenal IVC.
✔ In mega cava, the luminal diameter exceeds 28 mm. For adequate bilateral caval filtration, this condition requires bilateral placement of common iliac filters or a bird's nest filter (if the caval diameter is < 40 mm).
✔ Multiple right or left renal veins (including circumaortic) require placement of the legs of the filter below the lowest renal vein for adequate filtration. This eliminates the possibility of the formation of collateral venous pathways around the filter.
✘ Failure to diagnose anomalies of the renal veins and IVC places the patient at risk for inadequate DVT prophylaxis as well as complications of surgical procedures such as aortoiliac repair.
✘ IVC venography detects anomalies in 11% of patients, whereas selected renal venography detects anomalies in 37%.
✘ IVC venography via the right common femoral approach may fail to detect IVC duplication because the persistent left IVC typically drains into the left renal vein.

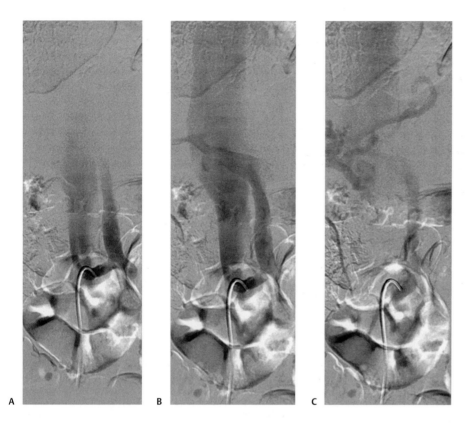

A   B   C

■ Clinical Presentation

The patient is a 57-year-old man previously treated for cirrhosis.

■ Imaging Findings

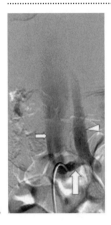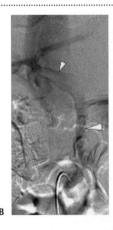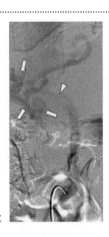

A   B   C

(A) Venography from a common femoral vein approach shows a patent inferior vena cava (IVC: *small arrow*) communicating via a short conduit (*large arrow*) with the superior mesenteric vein (SMV: *arrowhead*). **(B)** Delayed image shows a patent SMV (*large arrowhead*) and portal vein (PV: *small arrowhead*). **(C)** Further delayed image shows PV (*arrowhead*) and multiple mesenteric varices (*arrows*).

■ Differential Diagnosis

- **Mesocaval shunt:** Indicated by opacification of the SMV after injection of a vessel arising from the IVC.

■ Essential Facts

- Surgical portosystemic shunts include mesocaval, splenorenal, and portacaval types.
- Indications for surgical shunts are similar to those for transjugular intrahepatic portosystemic shunts (TIPS; see Case 58 for complete list). The principal indication is the treatment of complications related to portal hypertension.
- In general, TIPS placement is a less invasive and therefore a first-line method for creating a portosystemic shunt.
- Surgical shunts are reserved for patients for whom a TIPS is indicated but has failed or is not possible—including those with complete PV occlusion or extensive hepatic cysts.
- Surgical shunts have been created with side-to-side anastomoses as well as interposed synthetic or venous conduits. Venous conduits include internal jugular and external iliac veins.

■ Other Imaging Findings

- Venography may be the best option for the detection of complications related to surgical portosystemic shunts.
- Doppler ultrasound evaluation is more difficult with surgical shunts than with TIPS because of the absence of a solid organ window for ultrasonographic interrogation.

✔ Pearls & ✗ Pitfalls

- ✔ Of patients requiring a portosystemic shunt to treat complications of portal hypertension, 10% undergo surgical shunt creation and 90% undergo TIPS placement.
- ✗ Complications of surgical portosystemic shunts are similar to those of TIPS, including thrombosis, stenosis, and hepatic encephalopathy.
- ✗ Surgical portosystemic shunt thrombosis and stenosis can be treated by venoplasty and/or stent placement from the common femoral vein or internal jugular vein approach.

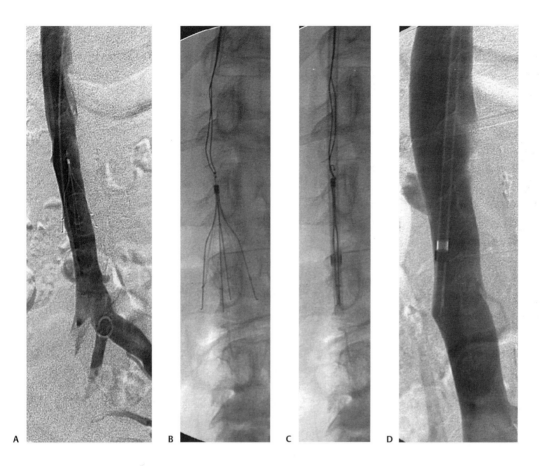

A   B   C   D

Clinical Presentation

The patient is a 53-year-old woman status post-knee replacement 8 weeks ago.

■ Imaging Findings

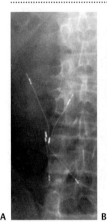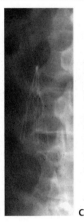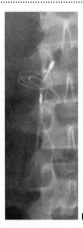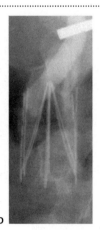

A   B   C   D

Case images on the previous page show removal of a Gunther Tulip (Cook Medical, Bloomington, IN) filter. Cavagram obtained before removal shows no intraluminal thrombus. The hook of the filter was successfully captured with a snare, the filter was resheathed, and a cavagram obtained after removal shows no caval rupture. Some permanent filters include **(A)** bird's nest (Cook Medical), **(B)** titanium Greenfield (Boston Scientific, Natick, MA), **(C)** Simon nitinol (CR Bard, Covington, GA), and **(D)** Vena Tech (B Braun Medical, Bethlehem, PA).

■ Differential Diagnosis

- *Inferior vena cava (IVC) filter placement and retrieval*

■ Essential Facts

- IVC filtration, or interruption, can be accomplished with two types of filters: permanent and removable.
- Removable filters may be temporary or optional.
- Temporary filters typically remain fixed to a delivery catheter and must be withdrawn when the catheter is removed.
- Optional filters may be left as permanent filters or retrieved. All removable filters marketed in the United States are of the optional type.
- Indications for IVC filters:
  - Deep venous thrombosis (DVT)/pulmonary embolism (PE) and contraindication to anticoagulation
  - DVT/PE and complication of anticoagulation
  - DVT/PE despite anticoagulation
  - Free-floating iliofemoral or IVC thrombus
  - Prophylaxis for patients at increased risk for PE/DVT and poor cardiopulmonary reserve
- Indications for removable IVC filters:
  - Before major surgery and extended immobility
  - After major trauma
  - In young patients with a long life expectancy and an indication for an IVC filter
- Indications for suprarenal IVC filters:
  - Renal vein, infrarenal or suprarenal caval thrombosis
  - Pregnancy
  - Recurrent PE despite IVC filter

■ Other Imaging Findings

- Venography is performed:
  - Before filter placement to assess caval diameter and location of the renal vein, and to detect any renal/IVC anomalies.
  - Before filter retrieval to assess for thrombus in the filter or IVC, filter fracture, or caval wall penetration.
  - After filter retrieval to rule out caval rupture.

✔ Pearls & ✘ Pitfalls

- ✔ Bird's nest filters are typically used when the caval diameter is > 28 mm (megacava). The diameter must be < 40 mm. Other than the bird's nest filter, most filters are designed for use when the caval diameter is < 28 mm.
- ✔ G2 Recovery filters (Bard) can be retrieved by capturing the apex with a cone retrieval apparatus and pulling them into a sheath.
- ✔ Celect (Cook) and Gunther Tulip filters can be retrieved by capturing an apical hook and oversheathing the filter. Limited captured thrombus (< 25% of filter volume) does not preclude removal.
- ✔ Slight apparent extension of the legs of a filter outside the confines of the IVC lumen on venography does not preclude filter removal (see first image of case).
- ✘ Complications of IVC filters include IVC or renal vein thrombosis, caval wall penetration, filter migration or fracture, and recurrent PE (2–7%).
- ✘ Extensive intraluminal thrombus within an optional filter may prevent retrieval. Thrombolysis may be an option.
- ✘ Alternative sources of PE include upper extremity veins, iliac veins (often incompletely imaged by ultrasound), renal veins, and gonadal veins. A superior vena cava filter or suprarenal IVC filter may be necessary.

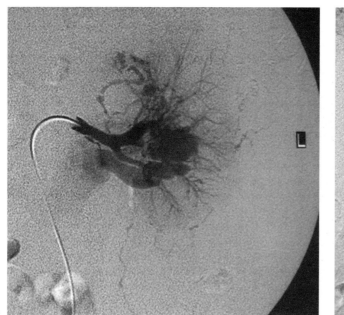
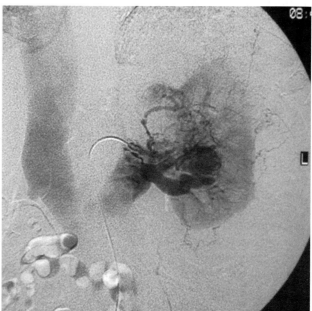

Clinical Presentation

The patient is a 59-year-old man who presented with left flank pain.

■ Imaging Findings

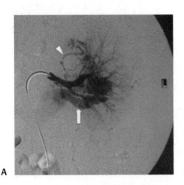 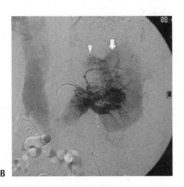 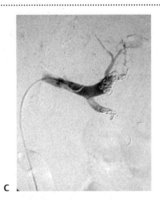

A   B   C

(A) Selected renal angiogram shows early opacification of the renal vein (*arrow*), dense neovascularity, and an ectatic capsular branch (*arrowhead*). **(B)** Delayed image shows renal nephrogram (*arrow*) and blush within an exophytic mass (*arrowhead*). **(C)** Capsular and parenchymal branches were embolized with Gelfoam and particles, and the anterior and posterior divisions of the renal artery were embolized with coils. The patient underwent nephrectomy the following day.

■ Differential Diagnosis

- ***Renal cell carcinoma (RCC):*** Suggested by arteriovenous (a-v) shunting, an exophytic mass, and dense neovascularity. RCC is commonly evaluated by conventional angiography with the intent to embolize or ablate before surgical resection.
- *Metastasis:* May cause neovascularity and shunting and should always be considered in the differential diagnosis of renal malignancy. Metastasis is uncommonly evaluated by conventional angiography.
- *Arteriovenous malformation:* Would have dense vascularity with shunting, but no neovascularity or exophytic mass.

■ Essential Facts

- RCC is usually extremely hypervascular and may invade adjacent structures, placing patients at risk for marked bleeding during surgical resection.
- Conventional angiography is performed with the intent to pretreat before surgical resection to markedly reduce intraoperative blood loss. Both primary RCC and metastases such as bone tumors can be pretreated.
- Other vascular masses of the kidney include adenomas, angiomyolipomas, oncocytomas, and metastases.
- Devascularization of the mass or kidney is accomplished by occluding the arterial supply, typically within 24 hours of surgical resection.
- Distal embolization minimizes persistent supply to the tumor by extensive collateral recruitment and may be accomplished with Gelfoam, polyvinyl alcohol, or tris-acryl particles.

- Alcohol ablation is an alternative. Absolute ethanol is injected while the renal artery is occluded with a balloon catheter to prevent nontarget ablation.
- Coil embolization of the main renal artery and its branches is adjunctive to distal embolization.
- Recruitment of atypical arterial feeders is common, including renal capsular branches and lumbar arteries. These branches may require presurgical embolization or ablation.

■ Other Imaging Findings

- Angiography for RCC shows intense neovascular blush, ectatic arterial supply to the tumor, a-v shunting, and venous thrombus.

✔ Pearls & ✗ Pitfalls

- ✔ Unlike RCC, oncocytomas, adenomas, and angiomyolipomas typically lack a-v shunting.
- ✔ Unlike RCC, oncocytomas may show a spoked wheel configuration to the arterial supply.
- ✗ Complications of interventional radiology therapies include tissue necrosis and infection, as well as nontarget embolization/ablation with ischemia.
- ✗ Before particle injection, a-v shunts may require coil embolization or the use of larger particles to prevent nontarget (pulmonary arterial) embolization.
- ✗ Coils placed at the origin of the renal artery can be dislodged during nephrectomy. Coils should be placed more distally or within the posterior and anterior divisions.

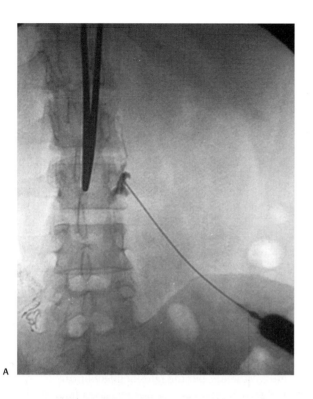

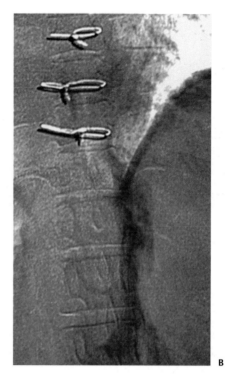

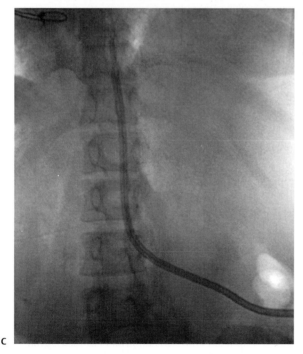

Clinical Presentation

A 60-year-old man with end-stage renal disease requires placement of a permanent catheter for hemodialysis.

■ Imaging Findings

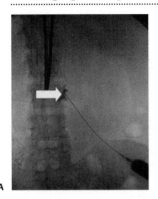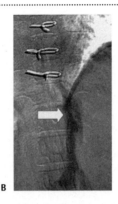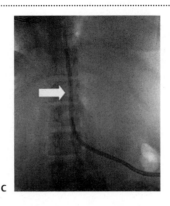

A   B   C

(A) Translumbar placement of a permanent hemodialysis catheter. With the patient prone, punctures are made to the right of the spine at L3 (*arrow*) from the level of the right iliac crest. **(B)** Contrast injection verifies direct inferior vena cava (IVC: *arrow*) puncture for permanent catheter placement. **(C)** Permanent catheter (*arrow*) is tunneled from the right side subcutaneously to the puncture site and advanced through a peel-away sheath until the tip is at the junction of the right atrium and IVC.

■ Differential Diagnosis

• ***Translumbar hemodialysis catheter***

■ Essential Facts

• For patients with end-stage renal disease treated with hemodialysis, the options for central venous access are gradually exhausted.
• The internal jugular veins are the first-line permanent access site for catheter placement because of a lower risk for procedural and delayed complications than at alternative sites.
• Alternative routes are used systematically after exhaustion of the jugular veins to minimize complications and maximize survival.
• Occluded jugular and small collateral veins can be recanalized as a second-line option.
• The subclavian veins are used next; they are avoided as a first option because of a higher rate of pneumothorax, stenosis, and thrombosis than when the internal jugular veins are used. Subclavian vein occlusion results in obstruction of the venous outflow of the arm and is associated with swelling, pain, and the loss of upper extremity arteriovenous shunt options.
• Alternatives to chest vein catheters include femoral, direct IVC, transhepatic, transrenal, and surgically placed direct right atrial catheters.
• Femoral catheters have a higher rate of infection and occlusion than chest catheters, resulting in more frequent

interventions for catheter maintenance. They may result in IVC occlusion.
• Translumbar IVC catheters malfunction more frequently than chest catheters, but the rates of infection are comparable.
• Transhepatic IVC or hepatic venous catheters have a high malfunction rate because of the constant movement of the catheter tip during respiratory excursion of the liver.
• Direct right atrial catheters can be placed surgically but do not allow over-the-wire catheter exchange.

✔ Pearls & ✘ Pitfalls

✔ Venous access sites for hemodialysis catheters should be used in a systematic, progressive manner to minimize complications and maximize survival.
✔ Catheter dysfunction should prompt thrombolytic infusion or over-the-wire catheter exchange before an alternative site is used.
✔ Mild catheter infections may respond to catheter exchange and antibiotics. Tract infection and sepsis typically require removal of permanent catheters and interim dialysis through temporary catheters.
✘ Complications of permanent catheter placement at any site include procedure-related complications such as pneumothorax, infection, bleeding, and nontarget puncture, injury, or catheterization, as well as delayed complications such as venous thrombosis, stenosis or occlusion, infection, and catheter malfunction.

Case 1

Creasy JD, Chiles C, Routh WD, Dyer RB. Overview of traumatic injury of the thoracic aorta. Radiographics 1997;17(1):27–45

Case 2

Alkadhi H, Wildermuth S, Desbiolles L, et al. Vascular emergencies of the thorax after blunt and iatrogenic trauma: multi-detector row CT and three-dimensional imaging. Radiographics 2004;24(5):1239–1255

Fisher RG, Sanchez-Torres M, Thomas JW, Whigham CJ. Subtle or atypical injuries of the thoracic aorta and brachiocephalic vessels in blunt thoracic trauma. Radiographics 1997;17(4):835–849

Case 3

Lockhart ME, Robbin ML. Case 58: giant cell arteritis. Radiology 2003;227(2):512–515

Case 4

Fava MP, Foradori GB, García CB, et al. Percutaneous transluminal angioplasty in patients with Takayasu arteritis: five-year experience. J Vasc Interv Radiol 1993;4(5):649–652

Gotway MB, Araoz PA, Macedo TA, et al. Imaging findings in Takayasu's arteritis. AJR Am J Roentgenol 2005;184(6):1945–1950

Case 5

Gonda RL Jr, Gutierrez OH, Azodo MV. Mycotic aneurysms of the aorta: radiologic features. Radiology 1988;168(2):343–346

Macedo TA, Stanson AW, Oderich GS, Johnson CM, Panneton JM, Tie ML. Infected aortic aneurysms: imaging findings. Radiology 2004;231(1):250–257

Case 6

Gutman H, Russo I, Neuman-Levin M, Haddad M, Zelikovski A. Computed tomography diagnosis of primary aorto-enteric fistula. Clin Imaging 1989;13(3):215–216

Hagspiel KD, Turba UC, Bozlar U, et al. Diagnosis of aortoenteric fistulas with CT angiography. J Vasc Interv Radiol 2007;18(4):497–504

Case 7

Hagspiel KD, Turba UC, Bozlar U, et al. Diagnosis of aortoenteric fistulas with CT angiography. J Vasc Interv Radiol 2007;18(4):497–504

Sharif MA, Lee B, Lau LL, et al. Prosthetic stent graft infection after endovascular abdominal aortic aneurysm repair. J Vasc Surg 2007;46(3):442–448

Case 8

Prasad S, Kasner SE. Teaching NeuroImage: subclavian steal syndrome. Neurology 2007;69(2):E1

Case 9

Gupta AK, Purkayastha S, Bodhey NK, Kapilamoorthy TR, Kesavadas C. Preoperative embolization of hypervascular head and neck tumours. Australas Radiol 2007;51(5):446–452

Case 10

Weaver FA, Comerota AJ, Youngblood M, et al. Surgical revascularization versus thrombolysis for non-embolic lower extremity native artery occlusions: results of a prospective randomized trial. J Vasc Surg 1996;24:513–521

Case 11

Albisetti M, Schmugge M, Haas R, et al. Arterial thromboembolic complications in critically ill children. J Crit Care 2005;20(3):296–300

Wang M, Hays T, Balasa V, et al; Pediatric Coagulation Consortium. Low-dose tissue plasminogen activator thrombolysis in children. J Pediatr Hematol Oncol 2003;25(5):379–386

Case 12

Rundback JH, Rozenblit GN, Poplausky MR. Renal artery stenting. In: Darcy MD, Vedantham S, Kaufman JA, eds. SCVIR Syllabus. Peripheral Vascular Interventions. 2nd ed. Fairfax, VA: Society of Cardiovascular and Interventional Radiology; 2001:279–293

van de Ven PJG, Kaatee R, Beutler JJ, et al. Arterial stenting and balloon angioplasty in ostial atherosclerotic renovascular disease: a randomised trial. Lancet 1999;353(9149):282–286

Case 13

Bakal CW, Cynamon J, Lakritz PS, Sprayregen S. Value of preoperative renal artery embolization in reducing blood transfusion requirements during nephrectomy for renal cell carcinoma. J Vasc Interv Radiol 1993;4(6):727–731

Mitchell SE, Shah AM, Schwengel D. Pulmonary artery pressure changes during ethanol embolization procedures to treat vascular malformations: can cardiovascular collapse be predicted? J Vasc Interv Radiol 2006;17(2 Pt 1):253–262

Case 14

De Gregorio MA, Gimeno MJ, Mainar A, et al. Mechanical and enzymatic thrombolysis for massive pulmonary embolism. J Vasc Interv Radiol 2002;13(2 Pt 1):163–169

Skaf E, Beemath A, Siddiqui T, Janjua M, Patel NR, Stein PD. Catheter-tip embolectomy in the management of acute massive pulmonary embolism. Am J Cardiol 2007;99(3):415–420

Case 15

Comerota AJ, Gravett MH. Iliofemoral venous thrombosis. J Vasc Surg 2007;46(5):1065–1076

Enden T, Sandvik L, Kløw NE, et al. Catheter-directed Venous Thrombolysis in acute iliofemoral vein thrombosis—the CaVenT study: rationale and design of a multicenter, randomized, controlled, clinical trial (NCT00251771). Am Heart J 2007;154(5):808–814

Case 16

Ferral H, Patel NH. Selection criteria for patients undergoing transjugular intrahepatic portosystemic shunt procedures: current status. J Vasc Interv Radiol 2005;16(4):449–455

Kang JY. Peptic ulcer in hepatic cirrhosis and renal failure. J Gastroenterol Hepatol 1994;9(Suppl 1):S20–S23

Case 17

Onal B, Ilgit ET, Koşar S, Akkan K, Gümüş T, Akpek S. Endovascular treatment of peripheral vascular lesions with stent-grafts. Diagn Interv Radiol 2005;11(3):170–174

Onal B, Koşar S, Gümüş T, Ilgit ET, Akpek S. Postcatheterization femoral arteriovenous fistulas: endovascular treatment with stent-grafts. Cardiovasc Intervent Radiol 2004;27(5):453–458

Case 18

Patel NH, Stookey KR, Ketcham DB, Cragg AH. Endovascular management of acute extensive iliofemoral deep venous thrombosis caused by May-Thurner syndrome. J Vasc Interv Radiol 2000;11(10):1297–1302

Case 19

d'Othée BJ, Haulon S, Mounier-Vehier C, Beregi JP, Jabourek O, Willoteaux S. Percutaneous endovascular treatment for stenoses and occlusions of infrarenal aorta and aortoiliac bifurcation: midterm results. Eur J Vasc Endovasc Surg 2002;24(6):516–523

Feugier P, Toursarkissian B, Chevalier JM, Favre JP; AURC. Endovascular treatment of isolated atherosclerotic stenosis of the infrarenal abdominal aorta: long-term outcome. Ann Vasc Surg 2003;17(4):375–385

Case 20

Eskandari MK, Brown KE, Kibbe MR, Morasch MD, Matsumura JS, Pearce WH. Restenosis after carotid stent placement in patients with previous neck irradiation or endarterectomy. J Vasc Interv Radiol 2007;18(11):1368–1374

Higashida RT, Meyers PM, Phatouros CC, Connors JJ III, Barr JD, Sacks D; Technology Assessment Committees of the American Society of Interventional and Therapeutic Neuroradiology and the Society of Interventional Radiology. Reporting standards for carotid artery angioplasty and stent placement. J Vasc Interv Radiol 2004;15(5):421–422

Case 21

Midgley PI, Mackenzie KS, Corriveau MM, et al. Blunt thoracic aortic injury: a single institution comparison of open and endovascular management. J Vasc Surg 2007;46(4):662–668

Perry MO. Complications of missed arterial injuries. J Vasc Surg 1993;17(2):399–407

Case 22

Chahwan S, Comerota AJ, Pigott JP, Scheuermann BW, Burrow J, Wojnarowski D. Elective treatment of abdominal aortic aneurysm with endovascular or open repair: the first decade. J Vasc Surg 2007;45(2):258–262, discussion 262

Eliason JL, Upchurch GR Jr. Endovascular abdominal aortic aneurysm repair. Circulation 2008;117(13):1738–1744

Case 23

Murad SD, Luong TK, Pattynama PM, Hansen BE, van Buuren HR, Janssen HL. Long-term outcome of a covered vs. uncovered transjugular intrahepatic portosystemic shunt in Budd-Chiari syndrome. Liver Int 2008;28(2):249–256

Panagiotou I, Kelekis DA, Karatza C, Nikolaou V, Mouyia V, Brountzos EN. Treatment of Budd-Chiari syndrome by transjugular intrahepatic portosystemic shunt. Hepatogastroenterology 2007; 54(78):1813–1816

Case 24

Lopera JE, Correa G, Brazzini A, et al. Percutaneous transhepatic treatment of symptomatic mesenteric venous thrombosis. J Vasc Surg 2002;36(5):1058–1061

Rodriguez-Luna H, Vargas HE. Portal vein thrombosis. Curr Treat Options Gastroenterol 2007;10(6):435–443

Case 25

Craig WD, Wagner BJ, Travis MD. Pyelonephritis: radiologic-pathologic review. Radiographics 2008;28(1):255–277, quiz 327–328

Lee WJ, Patel U, Patel S, Pillari GP. Emergency percutaneous nephrostomy: results and complications. J Vasc Interv Radiol 1994;5(1):135–139

Case 26

Mallery S, Freeman ML, Peine CJ, Miller RP, Stanchfield WR. Biliary-shunt fistula following transjugular intrahepatic portosystemic shunt placement. Gastroenterology 1996;111(5):1353–1357

Sze DY, Vestring T, Liddell RP, et al. Recurrent TIPS failure associated with biliary fistulae: treatment with PTFE-covered stents. Cardiovasc Intervent Radiol 1999;22(4):298–304

Case 27

Ferguson EC, Krishnamurthy R, Oldham SAA. Classic imaging signs of congenital cardiovascular abnormalities. Radiographics 2007;27(5):1323–1334

Tsai IC, Tzeng WS, Lee T, et al. Vertebral and carotid artery anomalies in patients with aberrant right subclavian arteries. Pediatr Radiol 2007;37(10):1007–1012

Case 28

Freedman AM, Sanyal AJ, Tisnado J, et al. Complications of transjugular intrahepatic portosystemic shunt: a comprehensive review. Radiographics 1993;13(6):1185–1210

Case 29

Srinivasaiah N, Reddy MS, Balupuri S, Talbot D, Jaques B, Manas D. Biliary cast syndrome: literature review and a single centre experience in liver transplant recipients. Hepatobiliary Pancreat Dis Int 2008;7(3):300–303

Starzl TE, Putnam CW, Hansbrough JF, Porter KA, Reid HA. Biliary complications after liver transplantation: with special reference to the biliary cast syndrome and techniques of secondary duct repair. Surgery 1977;81(2):212–221

Case 30

Chovanec V, Krajina A, Lojík M, Hůlek P, Vanásek T. TIPS creation in a patient with situs inversus totalis. Cardiovasc Intervent Radiol 2002;25(5):447–449

Postoak DW, Ferral H, Washburn WK, Speeg KV, Wholey MH. Transjugular intrahepatic portosystemic shunt creation in a patient with situs inversus. J Vasc Interv Radiol 2002;13(7):755–756

Case 31

Faust TW, Reddy KR. Postoperative jaundice. Clin Liver Dis 2004; 8(1):151–166

Park YS, Kim JH, Choi YW, et al. Percutaneous treatment of extrahepatic bile duct stones assisted by balloon sphincteroplasty and occlusion balloon. Korean J Radiol 2005;6(4):235–240

Case 32

Lamba M, Veinot JP, Acharya V, Moyana T. Fatal splenic arterial aneurysmal rupture associated with chronic pancreatitis. Am J Forensic Med Pathol 2002;23(3):281–283

Testart J, Boyet L, Perrier G, Clavier E, Peillon C. Arterial erosions in acute pancreatitis. Acta Chir Belg 2001;101(5):232–237, discussion 237–239

Case 33

Sajid MS, Ahmed N, Desai M, Baker D, Hamilton G. Upper limb deep vein thrombosis: a literature review to streamline the protocol for management. Acta Haematol 2007;118(1):10–18

Spence LD, Gironta MG, Malde HM, Mickolick CT, Geisinger MA, Dolmatch BL. Acute upper extremity deep venous thrombosis: safety and effectiveness of superior vena caval filters. Radiology 1999;210(1):53–58

Case 34

Castañeda-Zuniga WR, Jauregui H, Rysavy JA, Formanek A, Amplatz K. Complications of wedge hepatic venography. Radiology 1978;126(1):53–56

Semba CP, Saperstein L, Nyman U, Dake MD. Hepatic laceration from wedged venography performed before transjugular intrahepatic portosystemic shunt placement. J Vasc Interv Radiol 1996;7(1):143–146

Case 35

Patel NH, Jindal RM, Wilkin T, et al. Renal arterial stenosis in renal allografts: retrospective study of predisposing factors and outcome after percutaneous transluminal angioplasty. Radiology 2001;219(3):663–667

Case 36

Fan CM, Kaufman JA. Aortoiliac stenting: techniques and results. In: Darcy MD, Vedantham S, Kaufman JA, eds. SCVIR Syllabus. Peripheral Vascular Interventions. 2nd ed. Fairfax, VA: Society of Cardiovascular and Interventional Radiology; 2001:205–219

Case 37

Bandi R, Shetty PC, Sharma RP, Burke TH, Burke MW, Kastan D. Superselective arterial embolization for the treatment of lower gastrointestinal hemorrhage. J Vasc Interv Radiol 2001;12(12):1399–1405

Evangelista PT, Hallisey MJ. Transcatheter embolization for acute lower gastrointestinal hemorrhage. J Vasc Interv Radiol 2000;11(5):601–606

Case 38

Cho SK, Shin SW, Lee IH, et al. Balloon-occluded retrograde transvenous obliteration of gastric varices: outcomes and complications in 49 patients. AJR Am J Roentgenol 2007;189(6):W365–72

Case 39

Novellas S, Caramella T, Fournol M, Gugenheim J, Chevallier P. MR cholangiopancreatography features of the biliary tree after liver transplantation. AJR Am J Roentgenol 2008;191(1):221–227

Wojcicki M, Milkiewicz P, Silva M. Biliary tract complications after liver transplantation: a review. Dig Surg 2008;25(4):245–257

Case 40

Gillams A. Lung tumour ablation - where are we now? Cancer Imaging 2008;8:116–117

Zhu JC, Yan TD, Morris DL. A systematic review of radiofrequency ablation for lung tumors. Ann Surg Oncol 2008;15(6):1765–1774

Case 41

Ramchandani P, Cardella JF, Grassi CJ, et al; Society of Interventional Radiology Standards of Practice Committee. Quality improvement guidelines for percutaneous nephrostomy. J Vasc Interv Radiol 2003;14(9 Pt 2):S277–S281

Tuttle DN, Yeh BM, Meng MV, Breiman RS, Stoller ML, Coakley FV. Risk of injury to adjacent organs with lower-pole fluoroscopically guided percutaneous nephrostomy: evaluation with prone, supine, and multiplanar reformatted CT. J Vasc Interv Radiol 2005;16(11):1489–1492

Case 42

Aithal GP, Alabdi BJ, Rose JD, James OF, Hudson M. Portal hypertension secondary to arterio-portal fistulae: two unusual cases. Liver 1999;19(4):343–347

Dumortier J, Pilleul F, Adham M, et al. Severe portal hypertension secondary to arterio-portal fistula: salvage surgical treatment. Liver Int 2007;27(6):865–868

Case 43

Bloch R, Hoffer E, Borsa J, Fontaine A. Ehlers-Danlos syndrome mimicking mesenteric vasculitis: therapy, then diagnosis. J Vasc Interv Radiol 2001;12(4):527–529

Pepin M, Schwarze U, Superti-Furga A, Byers PH. Clinical and genetic features of Ehlers-Danlos syndrome type IV, the vascular type. N Engl J Med 2000;342(10):673–680

Case 44

Peterson JJ, Kransdorf MJ, Bancroft LW, Murphey MD. Imaging characteristics of cystic adventitial disease of the peripheral arteries: presentation as soft-tissue masses. AJR Am J Roentgenol 2003;180(3):621–625

Rai S, Davies RS, Vohra RK. Failure of endovascular stenting for popliteal cystic disease. Ann Vasc Surg 2009;23(3):410, e1–e5

Case 45

Browning PD, McGahan JP, Gerscovich EO. Percutaneous cholecystostomy for suspected acute cholecystitis in the hospitalized patient. J Vasc Interv Radiol 1993;4(4):531–537, discussion 537–538

Garcia-Sancho Tellez L, Rodriguez-Montes JA, Fernandez de Lis S, Garcia-Sancho Martin L. Acute emphysematous cholecystitis. Report of twenty cases. Hepatogastroenterology 1999;46(28):2144–2148

Case 46

Gossage JR, Kanj G. Pulmonary arteriovenous malformations. A state of the art review. Am J Respir Crit Care Med 1998;158(2):643–661

Pollak JS, Saluja S, Thabet A, Henderson KJ, Denbow N, White RI Jr. Clinical and anatomic outcomes after embolotherapy of pulmonary arteriovenous malformations. J Vasc Interv Radiol 2006;17(1):35–44, quiz 45

Case 47

Breyer BN, McAninch JW, Elliott SP, Master VA. Minimally invasive endovascular techniques to treat acute renal hemorrhage. J Urol 2008;179(6):2248–2252, discussion 2253

Manno C, Strippoli GF, Arnesano L, et al. Predictors of bleeding complications in percutaneous ultrasound-guided renal biopsy. Kidney Int 2004;66(4):1570–1577

Case 48

Rajan DK, Bunston S, Misra S, Pinto R, Lok CE. Dysfunctional autogenous hemodialysis fistulas: outcomes after angioplasty—are there clinical predictors of patency? Radiology 2004;232(2):508–515

Shatsky JB, Berns JS, Clark TWI, et al. Single-center experience with the Arrow-Trerotola Percutaneous Thrombectomy Device in the management of thrombosed native dialysis fistulas. J Vasc Interv Radiol 2005;16(12):1605–1611

Case 49

Berstad AE, Aabakken L, Smith HJ, Aasen S, Boberg KM, Schrumpf E. Diagnostic accuracy of magnetic resonance and endoscopic retrograde cholangiography in primary sclerosing cholangitis. Clin Gastroenterol Hepatol 2006;4(4):514–520

Weismüller TJ, Wedemeyer J, Kubicka S, Strassburg CP, Manns MP. The challenges in primary sclerosing cholangitis—aetiopatho-genesis, autoimmunity, management and malignancy. J Hepatol 2008;48(Suppl 1):S38–S57

Case 50

Basile A, Ragazzi S, Piazza D, Tsetis D, Lupattelli T, Patti MT. Hepatic artery pseudoaneurysm treated using stent-graft implantation and retrograde gastroduodenal artery coil embolization. Eur Radiol 2008;18(11):2579–2581

Tulsyan N, Kashyap VS, Greenberg RK, et al. The endovascular man-agement of visceral artery aneurysms and pseudoaneurysms. J Vasc Surg 2007;45(2):276–283, discussion 283

Case 51

Reilly LM, Ammar AD, Stoney RJ, Ehrenfeld WK. Late results follow-ing operative repair for celiac artery compression syndrome. J Vasc Surg 1985;2(1):79–91

Case 52

Landis MS, Rajan DK, Simons ME, Hayeems EB, Kachura JR, Snider-man KW. Percutaneous management of chronic mesenteric ischemia: outcomes after intervention. J Vasc Interv Radiol 2005;16(10):1319–1325

Rose SC, Quigley TM, Raker EJ. Revascularization for chronic mesen-teric ischemia: comparison of operative arterial bypass grafting and percutaneous transluminal angioplasty. J Vasc Interv Radiol 1995;6(3):339–349

Case 53

Bosch JL, Hunink MG. Meta-analysis of the results of percutaneous transluminal angioplasty and stent placement for aortoiliac occlu-sive disease. Radiology 1997;204(1):87–96

Cronenwett JL, Davis JT Jr, Gooch JB, Garrett HE. Aortoiliac occlusive disease in women. Surgery 1980;88(6):775–784

Case 54

Zeller T, Rastan A, Schwarzwälder U, et al. Midterm results after atherectomy-assisted angioplasty of below-knee arteries with use of the Silverhawk device. J Vasc Interv Radiol 2004;15(12):1391–1397

Case 55

Gaba RC, West DL, Bui JT, Owens CA, Marden FA. Covered stent treat-ment of carotid blowout syndrome. Semin Interv Radiol 2007;24(1):47–52

Case 56

Kato A, Kudo S, Matsumoto K, et al. Bronchial artery embolization for hemoptysis due to benign diseases: immediate and long-term results. Cardiovasc Intervent Radiol 2000;23(5):351–357

Mossi F, Maroldi R, Battaglia G, Pinotti G, Tassi G. Indicators predictive of success of embolisation: analysis of 88 patients with haemopty-sis. Radiol Med (Torino) 2003;105(1-2):48–55

Case 57

Inal M, Akgül E, Aksungur E, Demiryürek H, Yağmur O. Percutaneous self-expandable uncovered metallic stents in malignant biliary obstruction. Complications, follow-up and reintervention in 154 patients. Acta Radiol 2003;44(2):139–146

Isayama H, Komatsu Y, Tsujino T, et al. A prospective randomised study of "covered" versus "uncovered" diamond stents for the management of distal malignant biliary obstruction. Gut 2004;53(5):729–734

Lee BH, Choe DH, Lee JH, Kim KH, Chin SY. Metallic stents in malig-nant biliary obstruction: prospective long-term clinical results. AJR Am J Roentgenol 1997;168(3):741–745

Case 58

Ferral H. The evaluation of the patient undergoing an elective trans-jugular intrahepatic portosystemic shunt procedure. Semin Interv Radiol 2005;22:266–270

Case 59

Gonzalez-Juanatey C, Testa A, Vidan J, et al. Persistent left superior vena cava draining into the coronary sinus: report of 10 cases and literature review. Clin Cardiol 2004;27(9):515–518

Case 60

Spies JB, Ascher SA, Roth AR, Kim J, Levy EB, Gomez-Jorge J. Uter-ine artery embolization for leiomyomata. Obstet Gynecol 2001;98(1):29–34

Spies JB, Bruno J, Czeyda-Pommersheim F, Magee ST, Ascher SA, Jha RC. Long-term outcome of uterine artery embolization of leiomyo-mata. Obstet Gynecol 2005;106(5 Pt 1):933–939

Case 61

Hunink MG, Wong JB, Donaldson MC, Meyerovitz MF, de Vries J, Har-rington DP. Revascularization for femoropopliteal disease. A decision and cost-effectiveness analysis. JAMA 1995;274(2):165–171

Case 62

Sackett WR, Taylor SM, Coffey CB, et al. Ultrasound-guided thrombin in-jection of iatrogenic femoral pseudoaneurysms: a prospective analy-sis. Am Surg 2000;66(10):937–940, discussion 940–942

Case 63

Dethmers RS, Houpt P. Surgical management of hypothenar and the-nar hammer syndromes: a retrospective study of 31 instances in 28 patients. J Hand Surg [Br] 2005;30(4):419–4231

Ferris BL, Taylor LM Jr, Oyama K, et al. Hypothenar hammer syndrome: proposed etiology. J Vasc Surg 2000;31(1 Pt 1):104–113

Case 64

Kothary N, Soulen MC, Clark TWI, et al. Renal angiomyolipoma: long-term results after arterial embolization. J Vasc Interv Radiol 2005;16(1):45–50

Case 65

Antonello M, Frigatti P, Battocchio P, et al. Open repair versus endo-vascular treatment for asymptomatic popliteal artery aneurysm:

results of a prospective randomized study. J Vasc Surg 2005;
42(2):185–193

Case 66

Pollak JS, Saluja S, Thabet A, Henderson KJ, Denbow N, White RI Jr.
Clinical and anatomic outcomes after embolotherapy of pulmonary
arteriovenous malformations. J Vasc Interv Radiol 2006;17(1):35–
44, quiz 45

Case 67

Corbett HJ, Humphrey GME. Pulmonary sequestration. Paediatr Respir
Rev 2004;5(1):59–68
Curros F, Chigot V, Emond S, et al. Role of embolisation in the treatment of bronchopulmonary sequestration. Pediatr Radiol 2000;
30(11):769–773
Ko SF, Ng SH, Lee TY, et al. Noninvasive imaging of bronchopulmonary sequestration. AJR Am J Roentgenol 2000;175(4):1005–
1012

Case 68

Lorenz JM, Thomas JL. Complications of percutaneous fluid drainage.
Semin Interv Radiol 2006;23(2):194–204

Case 69

Divi V, Proctor MC, Axelrod DA, Greenfield LJ. Thoracic outlet decompression for subclavian vein thrombosis: experience in 71 patients.
Arch Surg 2005;140(1):54–57
Kreienberg PB, Chang BB, Darling RC III, et al. Long-term results in
patients treated with thrombolysis, thoracic inlet decompression,
and subclavian vein stenting for Paget-Schroetter syndrome. J Vasc
Surg 2001;33(2, Suppl)S100–S105

Case 70

Ryan JM, Suhocki PV, Smith TP. Coil embolization of segmental arterial mediolysis of the hepatic artery. J Vasc Interv Radiol 2000;
11(7):865–868
Sakano T, Morita K, Imaki M, Ueno H. Segmental arterial mediolysis
studied by repeated angiography. Br J Radiol 1997;70(834):656–
658

Case 71

Dinkel HP, Mettke B, Schmid F, Baumgartner I, Triller J, Do DD. Endovascular treatment of malignant superior vena cava syndrome: is
bilateral wallstent placement superior to unilateral placement? J
Endovasc Ther 2003;10(4):788–797

Case 72

Owen CC, Jain R. Acute acalculous cholecystitis. Curr Treat Options
Gastroenterol 2005;8(2):99–104

Case 73

Hyodoh H, Hori M, Akiba H, Tamakawa M, Hyodoh K, Hareyama
M. Peripheral vascular malformations: imaging, treatment ap-
proaches, and therapeutic issues. Radiographics 2005;25(Suppl 1):
S159–S171

Case 74

Zagol B, Book S, Krasuski RA. Late "adult form" scimitar syndrome
presenting with "infant form" complications. J Invasive Cardiol
2006;18(2):E82–E85

Case 75

Jacobowitz GR, Rosen RJ, Rockman CB, et al. Transcatheter embolization of complex pelvic vascular malformations: results and long-
term follow-up. J Vasc Surg 2001;33(1):51–55

Case 76

Baum RA, Carpenter JP, Golden MA, et al. Treatment of type 2 endoleaks after endovascular repair of abdominal aortic aneurysms:
comparison of transarterial and translumbar techniques. J Vasc
Surg 2002;35(1):23–29
Steinmetz E, Rubin BG, Sanchez LA, et al. Type II endoleak after
endovascular abdominal aortic aneurysm repair: a conservative
approach with selective intervention is safe and cost-effective. J
Vasc Surg 2004;39(2):306–313

Case 77

Lorenz JM, Blum M. Complications of percutaneous chest biopsy.
Semin Interv Radiol 2006;23(2):188–193
Richardson CM, Pointon KS, Manhire AR, Macfarlane JT. Percutaneous
lung biopsies: a survey of UK practice based on 5444 biopsies. Br J
Radiol 2002;75(897):731–735

Case 78

Levien LJ, Veller MG, Lambert AW. Popliteal artery entrapment
syndrome: more common than previously recognized. J Vasc Surg
1999;30(4):587–598
Stager A, Clement D. Popliteal artery entrapment syndrome. Sports
Med 1999;28(1):61–70

Case 79

Trigaux JP, Vandroogenbroek S, De Wispelaere JF, Lacrosse M, Jamart J.
Congenital anomalies of the inferior vena cava and left renal vein: evaluation with spiral CT. J Vasc Interv Radiol 1998;9(2):339–345

Case 80

Stavropoulos SW, Charagundla SR. Imaging techniques for detection
and management of endoleaks after endovascular aortic aneurysm
repair. Radiology 2007;243(3):641–655

Case 81

Darcy M. Treatment of lower gastrointestinal bleeding: vasopressin
infusion versus embolization. J Vasc Interv Radiol 2003;14(5):535–
543
Funaki B, Kostelic JK, Lorenz J, et al. Superselective microcoil embolization of colonic hemorrhage. AJR Am J Roentgenol 2001;
177(4):829–836

Case 82

Nealon WH, Walser E. Main pancreatic ductal anatomy can direct choice
of modality for treating pancreatic pseudocysts (surgery versus percutaneous drainage). Ann Surg 2002;235(6):751–758
Walser EM, Nealon WH, Marroquin S, Raza S, Hernandez JA, Vasek J.
Sterile fluid collections in acute pancreatitis: catheter drainage versus simple aspiration. Cardiovasc Intervent Radiol 2006;29(1):102–
107

Case 83

Davidson RA, Barri Y, Wilcox CS. Predictors of cure of hypertension
in fibromuscular renovascular disease. Am J Kidney Dis 1996;
28(3):334–3388

Surowiec SM, Sivamurthy N, Rhodes JM, et al. Percutaneous therapy for renal artery fibromuscular dysplasia. Ann Vasc Surg 2003;17(6):650–655

Case 84

Koops A, Wojciechowski B, Broering DC, Adam G, Krupski-Berdien G. Anatomic variations of the hepatic arteries in 604 selective celiac and superior mesenteric angiographies. Surg Radiol Anat 2004;26(3):239–244

Liu DM, Salem R, Bui JT, et al. Angiographic considerations in patients undergoing liver-directed therapy. J Vasc Interv Radiol 2005;16(7):911–935

Case 85

Velmahos GC, Toutouzas KG, Vassiliu P, et al. A prospective study on the safety and efficacy of angiographic embolization for pelvic and visceral injuries. J Trauma 2002;53(2):303–308, discussion 308

Case 86

Madoff DC, Wallace MJ, Ahrar K, Saxon RR. TIPS-related hepatic encephalopathy: management options with novel endovascular techniques. Radiographics 2004;24(1):21–36, discussion 36–37

Case 87

Altman DH, Puranik SR. Superior mesenteric artery syndrome in children. Am J Roentgenol Radium Ther Nucl Med 1973;118(1):104–108

Baltazar U, Dunn J, Floresguerra C, Schmidt L, Browder W. Superior mesenteric artery syndrome: an uncommon cause of intestinal obstruction. South Med J 2000;93(6):606–608

Case 88

Hood DB, Kuehne J, Yellin AE, Weaver FA. Vascular complications of thoracic outlet syndrome. Am Surg 1997;63(10):913–917

Case 89

Ciraulo DL, Luk S, Palter M, et al. Selective hepatic arterial embolization of grade IV and V blunt hepatic injuries: an extension of resuscitation in the nonoperative management of traumatic hepatic injuries. J Trauma 1998;45(2):353–358, discussion 358–359

Case 90

Kaminski A, Liu IL, Applebaum H, Lee SL, Haigh PI. Routine interval appendectomy is not justified after initial nonoperative treatment of acute appendicitis. Arch Surg 2005;140(9):897–901

Case 91

Slonim SM, Miller DC, Mitchell RS, Semba CP, Razavi MK, Dake MD. Percutaneous balloon fenestration and stenting for life-threatening ischemic complications in patients with acute aortic dissection. J Thorac Cardiovasc Surg 1999;117(6):1118–1126

Case 92

Tsolakis IA, Walvatne CS, Caldwell MD. Cystic adventitial disease of the popliteal artery: diagnosis and treatment. Eur J Vasc Endovasc Surg 1998;15(3):188–194

Case 93

Scultetus AH, Villavicencio JL, Gillespie DL. The nutcracker syndrome: its role in the pelvic venous disorders. J Vasc Surg 2001;34(5):812–819

Case 94

Stanson AW, Friese JL, Johnson CM, et al. Polyarteritis nodosa: spectrum of angiographic findings. Radiographics 2001;21(1):151–159

Case 95

Lambova SN, Kuzmanova SI. Raynaud's phenomenon in common rheumatic diseases. Folia Med (Plovdiv) 2006;48(3-4):22–28

Case 96

Hicks ME, Malden ES, Vesely TM, Picus D, Darcy MD. Prospective anatomic study of the inferior vena cava and renal veins: comparison of selective renal venography with cavography and relevance in filter placement. J Vasc Interv Radiol 1995;6(5):721–729

Trigaux JP, Vandroogenbroek S, De Wispelaere JF, Lacrosse M, Jamart J. Congenital anomalies of the inferior vena cava and left renal vein: evaluation with spiral CT. J Vasc Interv Radiol 1998;9(2):339–345

Case 97

Lorenz JM, Funaki B, Denison G. Balloon dilatation of a distal splenorenal shunt in a child. AJR Am J Roentgenol 2005;184(6):1915–1916

Orug T, Soonawalla ZF, Tekin K, Olliff SP, Buckels JA, Mayer AD. Role of surgical portosystemic shunts in the era of interventional radiology and liver transplantation. Br J Surg 2004;91(6):769–773

Case 98

Levy JM, Duszak RL Jr, Akins EW, et al. Inferior vena cava filter placement. American College of Radiology. ACR Appropriateness Criteria. Radiology 2000;215(Suppl):981–997

Case 99

Bakal CW, Cynamon J, Lakritz PS, Sprayregen S. Value of preoperative renal artery embolization in reducing blood transfusion requirements during nephrectomy for renal cell carcinoma. J Vasc Interv Radiol 1993;4(6):727–731

Case 100

Lorenz JM. Unconventional venous access techniques. Semin Interv Radiol 2006;23(3):279–286

Index

Note: Locators refer to case number. Locators in **boldface** indicate primary diagnosis.